Cornelia H. J. van der Ziel, MD, FACOG, is a practicing staff obstetrician and gynecologist working for Harvard Vanguard Medical Associates in Cambridge, Massachusetts. She is a clinical instructor in obstetrics and gynecology at Harvard Medical School, with special interests in high-risk obstetrics, adolescent medical issues, and menopause. The author emigrated with her family from the Netherlands as a young child and now lives in Brookline, Massachusetts, with her family.

Jacqueline Tourville is a certified childbirth educator and holds advanced degrees in history and education. Born in the Adirondacks region of New York State, Jacqueline currently resides in New Hampshire with her husband and daughter.

D0826896

big,
beautiful
pregnant

EXPERT ADVICE AND COMFORTING WISDOM FOR THE
EXPECTING PLUS-SIZE WOMAN

big,
beautiful
pregnant

CORNELIA VAN DER ZIEL, MD,
AND JACQUELINE TOURVILLE

MARLOWE & COMPANY
NEW YORK

BIG, BEAUTIFUL AND PREGNANT:
Expert Advice and Comforting Wisdom for the Expecting Plus-Size Woman

Copyright © 2006 by Cornelia van der Ziel and Jacqueline Tourville

Published by
Marlowe & Company
An Imprint of Avalon Publishing Group, Incorporated
245 West 17th Street • 11th floor
New York, NY 10011

Library of Congress Cataloging-in-Publication Data

Van der Ziel, Cornelia.
Expert advice and comforting wisdom for the expecting plus-size woman
/ Cornelia van der Ziel and Jacqueline Tourville.
p. cm.
Includes index.
ISBN 1-56924-319-0 (pbk.)
1. Pregnancy—Popular works. 2. Overweight women—Health and
hygiene—Popular works. I. Tourville, Jacqueline. II. Title.
RG525.V328 2006
618.2'4—dc22
2006007832

ISBN-13: 978–1-56924–319–0

Designed by Pauline Neuwirth, Neuwirth & Associates, Inc.

Printed in the United States of America

To my children, the raising of whom has taught me more about interpersonal relationships than I ever learned in school
—CV

To Jason and Claire, with much love
—JT

CONTENTS

FOREWORD

CONGRATULATIONS ON YOUR pregnancy! These next nine months promise to be an exciting time as you prepare for your child's birth. Based on what my overweight patients have shared with me, I know that your anticipation is accompanied by quite a few weight-related questions and concerns. You want to know what steps you can take to make your plus-size pregnancy the healthiest possible experience.

Research shows that, as a group, plus-size women are at higher risk for developing certain complications such as gestational diabetes and gestational hypertension. What happens during an individual plus-size woman's pregnancy, however, is based largely on her personal health choices and previous medical history. If you were generally healthy before becoming pregnant, carefully monitor diet and exercise, and actively participate in your prenatal care, you will likely have a healthy pregnancy.

The best way to gain valuable information about your own plus-size pregnancy is to attend all prenatal appointments and ask your obstetrician or midwife the questions you want answered. In between checkups, I recommend you do everything in your power to educate yourself about pregnancy and childbirth. Read pregnancy books, watch childbirth videos, and attend prenatal classes. Take advantage of every opportunity to learn about this unique life experience.

Until now, it has been difficult for plus-size women to find resources that adequately address weight-related pregnancy issues. Even with current statistics showing that more than half of all childbearing age women in the United States are considered overweight or obese, most pregnancy books contain minimal information about plus-size pregnancy. Because understanding your pregnancy is so central to taking good care of yourself, a book like this is long overdue.

No one claims being overweight and pregnant is easy. You must pay close attention to proper diet and exercise, follow your prenatal care provider's weight-gain guidelines, and possibly be prepared for a few extra tests to make sure both you and your baby are doing just fine. Closely working with your obstetrician or midwife and reading about pregnancy in books like this one demonstrate you are clearly on your way to achieving the healthiest possible pregnancy and childbirth experience. While the next nine months may present its own share of challenges, always remember that you pregnancy is an event to be cherished and honored.

—Cornelia van der Ziel, MD

INTRODUCTION

A Pregnancy Book Just for You!

THIS BOOK IS for every plus-size woman who has read other pregnancy guides only to think, *What about me? What steps should I take to make my pregnancy healthy and happy?* With growing numbers of women entering pregnancy already above their ideal weight, we decided it was time to write a different kind of pregnancy book. One not meant to chastise, scare, or ignore women because of their size, but a resource designed to provide plus-size women with accurate and balanced information. We hope *Big, Beautiful and Pregnant* finally gives you what you have been looking for—sound advice, reassurance, and, most of all, a sense of belonging.

What to Expect When You're Reading This Book

AS COAUTHORS, WE bring two very different perspectives to plus-size pregnancy. One of us is an obstetrician who has cared for countless plus-size patients, and the other is a woman who became pregnant just as her weight reached an all-time high. You will probably notice these distinct viewpoints as you read along. Some chapters are written directly from Jacqueline's own plus-size experience: "The Sisterhood's Guide to Prenatal Health Care" presents a candid look at the medical

1

ACCEPT YOURSELF:
Key Steps to a Healthy Pregnancy

The Journey Begins

My plan was always: (1) Lose weight (2) Get pregnant. I looked at the home pregnancy test and two parallel purple lines told me my master plan was now out the window. I was pregnant, or more correctly, plus-sized and pregnant. Something I had never prepared for or anticipated. I was elated at the thought of having a baby, but my weight problem hung like a black cloud over my excitement. What could I expect from plus-size pregnancy? I had no idea.

—JACQUELINE, age 29

WHETHER YOUR PLUS-SIZE pregnancy is a complete surprise or the result of calculated efforts to conceive, whether you are expecting your first child or your fourth, whether you weigh 16 or 60 pounds too much, the starting point for a healthy, successful plus-size pregnancy is simple . . .

Accept yourself. For at least these next nine months, take a break from crash diets and yo-yo weight loss. Put aside feelings of self-judgment if you don't quite look like the models in the pregnancy magazines. Few women actually do. Concentrate instead on taking excellent care of yourself. Enjoy every minute of your uniquely beautiful pregnancy. Allow yourself to excitedly prepare for the birth of your child. Learn to trust and love your body again—or for the first time. It is performing miraculous work.

Pregnancy is a journey and, just like going on any trip, it's always better to know where you are headed. This chapter outlines key steps you can take NOW to point your plus-size pregnancy in the right direction. You will learn what a measurement called *body mass index* can tell you about your pregnancy; why you should compile your personal and family medical history; how excellent nutrition, safe exercise, and a positive self-image can maximize your health and your baby's well-being; and where to find support for the issues you may face as a plus-size woman. For those of you reading this and are just beginning to ponder the possibility of becoming pregnant, we offer sensible information about your preconception weight.

You will hear the voices of many big, beautiful, and pregnant women sprinkled throughout this chapter. The sisters are here to share a few stories and tips of their own for making your pregnancy exactly what it should be: the adventure of a lifetime.

Educate Yourself

I began reading all the usual pregnancy books and, much to my frustration, I quickly realized plus-size women generally received two mentions in most books— one at the beginning where it said to lose weight before conceiving and the other in the section on gestational diabetes. In some books, plus-size pregnancy wasn't even mentioned. In all my reading I never really found specific advice for how a plus-size woman can take better care of herself and her growing baby.

—JACQUELINE, age 29

UNDERSTANDING HOW TO best care for your plus-size pregnancy begins with evaluating how healthy you are as your pregnancy begins. This is accomplished by compiling your personal and family medical/health history and determining a number called body mass index.

Body Mass Index

The medical community fortunately realizes something you already know—that you are much more than just a number on your bathroom scale. Body mass index (BMI) is a measurement you and your provider can use to estimate how much weight you should gain over the course of your pregnancy and evaluate your risk for possibly encountering certain complications. Instead of simply measuring the pull of gravity on your body (like a scale), BMI looks at the ratio between your weight and *height*. BMI honors the difference between a five-foot-tall woman who weighs 200 pounds and a six-foot-tall woman who weighs the same amount.

BMI is calculated by dividing your prepregnancy weight (in kilograms) by the square of your height (in meters). Your prepregnancy weight is used because your weight at this time is still just you! The chart on page 10 lets you easily determine your prepregnancy BMI.

Your height/weight ratio falls into one of the following categories:

Normal Weight: BMI between 20 and 24.9
Overweight: BMI between 25 and 29.9
Obese: BMI above 30

BMI is primarily used as a guideline for healthy pregnancy weight gain. This is the amount of weight you should gain to ensure your baby is getting all the nutrients needed for optimal growth and development. The Institute of Medicine endorses the following recommendations for total weight gain during pregnancy:

Normal BMI: weight gain between 25 and 35 pounds
Overweight BMI: weight gain between 15 and 25 pounds
Obese BMI: weight gain of at least 15 pounds

It is important to note that plus-size women pregnant with twins, triplets, or more have very different pregnancy weight gain goals. Your prenatal care provider can help you determine the ideal weight gain for your individual needs.

BMI is also used to evaluate your risk for *possibly* encountering complications during pregnancy (along with personal and family health history, as described in the following section). The majority of plus-size women have perfectly normal pregnancies and healthy babies. However, certain pregnancy-related problems, such as gestational hypertension and gestational diabetes (pregnancy-only forms of high blood pressure and diabetes) do occur more frequently in women with an obese BMI and, to a lesser extent, an overweight BMI. You will read much more about the health issues associated with plus-size pregnancy throughout this book.

Uncover Your Personal and Family Health History

BMI is a very useful tool, but is unable to explain something very simple. How can two plus-size women with identical weights and heights

Body Mass Index Table

	Normal					Overweight					Obese																
BMI	20	21	22	23	24	25	26	27	28	29	30	31	32	33	34	35	36	37	38	39	40	41	42	43	44	45
Height (inches)	Body weight (pounds)																									
58	95	100	105	110	115	120	124	129	134	139	144	148	153	158	163	167	172	177	182	187	191	196	201	206	211	215
59	99	104	109	114	119	124	128	133	138	143	148	153	158	163	168	173	178	183	188	193	198	203	208	213	218	223
60	102	107	112	118	123	128	133	138	143	148	153	158	163	168	174	179	184	189	194	199	204	209	215	220	225	230
61	106	111	116	122	127	132	137	143	148	153	158	164	169	174	180	185	190	195	201	206	211	217	222	227	232	238
62	109	115	120	126	131	136	142	147	153	158	164	169	175	180	186	191	196	202	207	213	218	224	229	235	240	246
63	113	118	124	130	135	141	146	152	158	163	169	175	180	186	191	197	203	208	214	220	225	231	237	242	248	254
64	117	122	128	134	140	145	151	157	163	169	174	180	186	192	197	204	209	215	221	227	232	238	244	250	256	262
65	120	126	132	138	144	150	156	162	168	174	180	186	192	198	204	210	216	222	228	234	240	246	252	258	264	270
66	124	130	136	142	148	155	161	167	173	179	186	192	198	204	210	216	223	229	235	241	247	253	260	266	272	278
67	128	134	140	146	153	159	166	172	178	185	191	198	204	211	217	223	230	236	242	249	255	261	268	274	280	287
68	132	138	144	151	158	164	171	177	184	190	197	203	210	216	223	230	236	243	249	256	262	269	276	282	289	295
69	135	142	149	155	162	169	176	182	189	196	203	209	216	223	230	236	243	250	257	263	270	277	284	291	297	304
70	139	146	153	160	167	174	181	188	195	202	207	216	222	229	236	243	250	257	264	271	278	285	292	299	306	313
71	143	150	157	165	172	179	186	193	200	208	215	222	229	236	243	250	257	265	272	279	286	293	301	308	315	322
72	147	154	162	169	177	184	191	199	206	213	221	228	235	242	250	258	265	272	279	287	294	302	309	316	324	331
73	152	159	166	174	182	189	197	204	212	219	227	235	242	250	257	265	272	280	288	295	302	310	318	325	333	340
74	156	164	171	179	186	194	202	210	218	225	233	241	249	256	264	272	280	287	295	303	311	319	326	334	342	350

experience completely different pregnancy outcomes? Predicting what to expect over the next nine months requires a more detailed picture of your pregnancy than one offered by your BMI alone. This means taking a closer look at your personal and family health history.

What information do you need to uncover? Anything that will help you and your provider identify potential trouble spots for your pregnancy. It is best to do this before conceiving, but it is never too late to find out what you need to know to put your pregnancy on the right track. Answering the following questions should help get your health inventory started:

- **What is the state of your general health?** Are you in reasonably good shape? Have you had any medical problems in the past? Have you ever had surgery? What for? Do you have high blood pressure? When was the last time you had your blood sugar checked? Plus-size women entering pregnancy with certain medical conditions, such as chronic hypertension (high blood pressure) or diabetes, require extra care and must work closely with their prenatal care providers for best results.
- **Do you take any medications on a regular basis?** Always check with your provider to make sure your medications are safe. Some prescribed drugs (such as ACE inhibitors for high blood pressure) may harm a developing fetus. Your provider can prescribe a pregnancy-safe alternative or advise you how to manage your condition through diet and/or exercise.
- **Do you smoke?** Cigarettes are always a bad idea but are especially dangerous for you and your baby during pregnancy. Cigarette smoking restricts the flow of blood through your blood vessels, reducing the level of oxygen and nutrients reaching your baby. Babies are more likely to develop intrauterine growth restriction (IUGR), a serious health problem. Smokers are more likely to have a baby born with a birth defect, for instance, a cleft palate and/or cleft lip. Women who smoke are also more likely to have a miscarriage. If you ever needed motivation to kick the habit, this is it. Talk to your health care provider or contact your hospital's community outreach center to find out what smoking cessation programs and support groups are available in your area.
- **What health problems run in your family?** If close family members, male or female, have high blood pressure or diabetes, you may be genetically predisposed to these disorders.

Because pregnancy is a time of increased physical stress, it is not uncommon for symptoms to appear at this time. Gestational diabetes, gestational hypertension, and preeclampsia (a related form of gestational hypertension) all occur more frequently in women with inherited tendencies for these conditions. Some investigating on your part may be necessary if you are uncertain about your family's medical history.

- **Have any family members experienced problems with their pregnancies?** Many complications encountered by either mother or fetus have some genetic link. Ask women in your family to describe their pregnancy and childbirth experiences. If these conversations reveal a particular health problem runs in your family, be sure to mention it to your prenatal care provider.

- **What were your previous pregnancies like?** If you have been pregnant before, did you carry the pregnancy to term? Was it an "easy" pregnancy? If not, what was the problem? Did you deliver vaginally or by cesarean section? Even if you weighed less during your other pregnancies, your previous experience is often the best indicator of what you can expect right now.

Every plus-size woman and every plus-size pregnancy is unique. Your personal and family health history, along with your BMI, enables you and your prenatal care provider to formulate a custom-fit plan for taking excellent care of your pregnancy.

Eat Right

Before becoming pregnant, my first waking thought on most mornings was "Today I start losing weight!" I tried everything from Weight Watchers to Atkins to pure starvation. I lost sixty pounds and gained back eighty. I then lost and gained the same twenty pounds about five times. Riding this diet roller coaster took its toll. I mistrusted my body and doubted my own willpower. I trained myself to dislike what I saw in the mirror. I put off buying new clothes until I could lose ten, then twenty, and then thirty pounds. I was unhappy if the number on the scale went up, happy if it went down.

My pregnancy gave me the chance to finally get off the diet roller coaster and make peace with myself. I started eating a wide variety of healthy foods, not because it was the latest fad diet or promised to make me lose ten pounds in a week, but because the foods were good for me and good for my baby. Eating with a healthy pregnancy as my motivation, and not fitting into the jeans I wore in high school, made it almost too easy to make the right choices. When I gave birth to a beautiful, healthy baby girl I felt like a completely different person than the woman who doubted her body could even become pregnant.

—JACQUELINE, age 29

YEARS ON THE diet roller coaster may have left you, like Jacqueline, unsure of what "eating right" even entails. Embrace your pregnancy as a chance to rediscover the pleasure of eating a healthy, balanced diet. Nutrients from the foods you eat are the building blocks for your baby's growth and development. Provide your baby with excellent nutrition from the very beginning. What you eat for the next nine months also matters for your own health. Nutrient-dense food choices help your body adjust better to the physical stress of being pregnant and may decrease how likely you are to encounter certain pregnancy problems.

So, what should you eat? Your pregnancy menu plan should be packed with a wide variety of fruits, vegetables, and whole grains, as well as healthy sources of protein and fats. Choose foods rich in vitamins and minerals. The very real benefits of eating a nutritious, balanced diet during pregnancy are numerous:

- Well-nourished women have lower rates of preeclampsia. Eating a well-rounded diet, especially rich in vitamins C and E, may prevent this complication.
- Eating a wide variety of nutritious foods enables you to better control pregnancy weight gain. Why? A turkey sandwich with lettuce, tomato, and mayonnaise on whole wheat bread, one cup of soup, a granola bar, and an apple for lunch will leave you feeling full a lot longer and will provide you with more nutrients than would a cheeseburger, soda, and fries from any fast-food outlet. Both these lunches have about the same number of calories.
- Iron is an important mineral both you and your baby rely on for red blood cell production. You need 27 mg of iron each day during pregnancy. Iron in your diet comes from many sources, including spinach, iron-fortified breads and cereals, and meat. You store reserves of iron in your body. Shortly before birth, your baby creates his or her own mineral storehouse. If you do not consume enough iron (through diet or supplementation),

you run an increased risk for developing iron-deficiency anemia. Eating iron-rich foods throughout pregnancy helps replenish your iron stores, enhances red blood cell production, and prevents anemia.

- Folic acid, a B vitamin contained in fortified grains and cereals and naturally found as folate in dark leafy green vegetables and fruit, helps to prevent serious birth defects such as spina bifida. You need at least 400 micrograms (mcg) of folic acid every day. According to the Centers for Disease Control, two-thirds of women in the United States do not get enough of this important vitamin. Because neural tube defects occur very early on in pregnancy, sometimes before you even realize you have missed your period, start filling your diet with foods rich in folate/folic acid, and take a daily prenatal vitamin with folic acid or a multivitamin with 400 mcg folic acid for at least one month before you conceive.

- For many plus-size women diagnosed with gestational diabetes, controlling the complication is often achieved through diet alone. The "diabetic diet" is simply a healthy, balanced diet with a little more attention paid to the number and type of carbohydrates consumed during each meal and snack. See chapter 7 for more information about gestational diabetes.

- Omega-3 fatty acids, found in foods such as walnuts, salmon, flaxseed, and enriched eggs, boost your baby's brain and eye development, improve your cholesterol levels, and reduce your overall risk for heart disease.

- Consuming at least 1,000 mg of calcium each day lowers your risk for developing osteoporosis later in life. If you do not get enough calcium in your diet (or through calcium supplements), your body does the generous thing and uses calcium from your own bones to make your baby's bones stronger. Drinking four cups of milk each day will provide you with your daily calcium requirement. One cup of milk averages about 300 mg of calcium.

Nutritious eating during pregnancy usually requires making only simple modifications most women can easily manage. You probably won't need to completely overhaul your current eating habits or give up your favorite foods in order to achieve the results described above. Please read chapter 5, "Prenatal Nutrition," for everything you need to know about how to construct a healthy prenatal diet.

Exercise

During my first pregnancy, I never exercised. While my blood pressure and blood sugar were both fine, I felt tired and washed out for pretty much the entire nine months. The second time around I changed my habits and began walking for a half-hour every day. Even though I weighed more than before and spent my days chasing around after a busy toddler, I felt energetic and alive. It was that simple.

—SARAH, age 34

REGULAR PHYSICAL ACTIVITY during pregnancy can strengthen muscle tone, enhance your cardiovascular health, relieve stress and anxiety, boost your energy levels, and burn off excess calories—helping you better meet pregnancy weight-gain goals. Exercise is a pregnancy problem solver. Women who exercise throughout pregnancy complain less frequently of constipation, hip and back pain, leg cramps, and trouble sleeping. Some women with gestational diabetes can actually control the disorder through exercise.

If all this information has got you pumped, great! Just remember to talk with your prenatal care provider about whether or not exercise is beneficial for your pregnancy. Exercise is not safe for all pregnancies and your provider's approval is necessary before embarking on *any* prenatal fitness program.

Once you get the okay from your provider, take stock of your physical fitness. Were you regularly exercising before pregnancy? If not, the key to successfully incorporating physical activity into your daily routine is to start slow. Walking for ten to twenty minutes a few times a week is often the best way to begin. Work your way up from there with whatever feels good for your body. Always stop exercising if you feel pain or shortness of breath.

Women who regularly worked out before becoming pregnant might be able to continue with their usual activities by making minor modifications such as not taking part in activities requiring any jumping up and down (like high impact aerobics) and, after the twentieth week of pregnancy, staying off their back while exercising.

For safe and healthy pregnancy exercises for plus-size women of all fitness levels see chapter 6, "Prenatal Exercise."

Find Support

We told my extended family about my pregnancy while visiting my aunt's house on Thanksgiving. Everyone was ecstatic. After dinner I chatted with my cousin who told me all about her own pregnancy and childbirth experiences. Unlike my skinny and petite sisters, Marie looked just like me—tall and big-boned. She had uncomplicated pregnancies with all three of her children and gave birth each time without medical intervention.

When the subject of weight came up, I'll never forget Marie's reassuring words, "Maybe it would have been better if you had lost some weight before becoming pregnant, but here's what's important right now. You're a strong, healthy woman who comes from a long line of strong, healthy women. Take good care of yourself and—no matter what—don't question your ability to have a successful pregnancy." Forget the turkey and the stuffing, talking to my cousin was what I was most grateful for that Thanksgiving. Her encouragement was exactly what I needed.

I kept in constant contact with my cousin throughout the rest of my pregnancy and our frequent conversations never failed to provide me with comfort and insight. It was a relief to talk to another plus-size woman who knew exactly what I was going through. I found it deeply inspiring to know another member of my family was so firmly in my corner.

—JACQUELINE, age 29

EVERY PLUS-SIZE woman deserves to feel supported in her efforts to take good care of herself and her unborn child. Surround yourself with nurturing people who will assist you in making healthy choices for your pregnancy. Seek guidance from those who will truly listen to your fears and anxiety and be able to provide sound advice.

Strong pregnancy support networks can consist of many familiar faces and quite a few brand new acquaintances:

- **Your family and friends:** Your first line of support comes from the people closest to you. Enlist your family's help to plan healthy meals. Take a nightly walk with your partner or a good friend. Especially if you are expecting your first child, make sure your partner learns about pregnancy right along with you. Attend prenatal classes together to find out more about prenatal nutrition and fitness, birthing options, newborn care, and breastfeeding. Have your partner read this book! When pregnancy becomes something you both share (or your entire family if you already have children), it helps to know someone else is rooting for your success.

- **Your prenatal care provider:** Whether you see an OB, midwife, or a family practitioner, your prenatal care provider understands that plus-size pregnancy can carry with it increased anxiety and worry. Maximize your provider's ability to take excellent care of your pregnancy by being open with your concerns. Your provider can help you locate community resources (support groups, prenatal classes) or refer you to other medical professionals who specialize in the issues you need addressed. You may see a nutritionist to assist with meal planning or a counselor/therapist to help you cope with emotional concerns.

  Because your prenatal care plays such a crucial role in your pregnancy, we have a whole chapter devoted to the subject. Please read chapter 3, "Guide to Prenatal Health Care," for more information.

- **Plus-size women:** Who else knows what a struggle it is just to find decent plus-size maternity clothes? Who else shares your same fears and anxieties? Connecting with other plus-size pregnant women is a powerful way to let you know you are not alone. Finding support from other plus-size women might be as easy as picking up the phone and calling your sister, your cousin, a co-worker, or a good friend. Or maybe the people in your immediate circle of friends and family are loving and encouraging, but just have not walked in your shoes. If that's the case, don't worry, the plus-size and pregnant crowd is easily accessible.

  Where can you find other women like yourself? The Internet is a great place to start. Major pregnancy Web sites contain moderated plus-size pregnancy message boards. If you feel lonely or isolated, participating in vibrant discussions about the very topics you most want to know about can provide welcome relief. See "Resources," for Web site addresses.

  Another option doesn't require a computer. Check with your provider or local hospital to see if any weight-related pregnancy support groups are offered in your community. Some groups will probably be geared for pregnant women with eating disorders, but there may be groups solely devoted to plus-size pregnancy. If your community does not offer a relevant support group for plus-size women, why not be brave and start one?

Feeling supported—that others truly care about you and the out-come of your pregnancy—helps you relax and enjoy a renewed sense of confidence in your body's ability to nourish and grow a baby.

DOMESTIC VIOLENCE

SOME WOMEN, unfortunately, experience the opposite of a supported preg-nancy. Approximately 1 in 20 pregnant women is a victim of domestic violence. If you can answer yes to any of the following questions, the National Domestic Violence Hotline urges you to seek help at once:

- Are you ever afraid of or intimidated by your partner?
- Does your partner try to isolate and control your actions by not letting you see certain family members and friends?
- Do you need to ask permission from your partner before leaving the house? Does your partner demand you return at a certain time or face the consequences?
- Has your partner ever threatened to harm you or your unborn baby?
- Has your partner pushed or hit you, thrown things at you, or forced you to have sex?
- Does your partner act like the abuse is no big deal or is your fault?

Women in abusive relationships experience a wide range of emotions—shame, fear, guilt, anger, or hopelessness. Don't make excuses for domestic violence. Talk with somebody you trust about your situation: a friend or relative, your pre-natal care provider, a co-worker, or someone in your religious community. Gather together an "emergency kit" of essentials—identification, keys, prenatal vita-mins, medications, phone card, money—in case you need to leave home on short notice. Call the National Domestic Violence Hotline at 1-800-799-SAFE (1-800-799-7233) to find out about shelters and programs for abused women in your area. Call 911 if you are in immediate danger. Reach out for the support and assistance you and your unborn baby deserve.

Feel Good about Yourself

Besides a healthy baby, what gifts did my plus-size pregnancy give me? Finally loving the person I saw when I looked in the mirror. Realizing my body, so com-petently growing another living being, deserved kindness and respect. Recognizing that beauty comes in all shapes and sizes—even a curvy, full-figured pregnant woman like me.

—KENDRA, age 27

WOMEN ARE CONSTANTLY bombarded with media images telling us that unless we fit into a size 4, we are not good-looking, sexy, smart, healthy, or worthy of love. Reject these warped messages. Self-accept-ance and a positive self-image—feeling good about your body regard-less of weight or dress size—makes deciding to take excellent care of your pregnancy a much easier choice. If body image is an issue you struggle with as a plus-size woman, the following strategies can help you feel good about the skin you are in:

- **Acknowledge your beauty.** Look in the mirror and lovingly take note of how your pregnant body transforms as the weeks and months pass—your curves grow curvier, your breasts become fuller, your belly swells. Delight in these physical changes. Recognize that these are outward signs of your baby's presence and your body's powerful preparations for birth and motherhood. Tell yourself that you are beautiful. Believe this statement.
- **Change your self-talk.** If your inner voice tends to be neg-ative, consciously insert more positive thoughts. Compliment yourself when you take the time to eat a nutritious lunch, remind yourself how wonderful it is that you went for a walk every day for the past week, congratulate yourself on doing a great job being pregnant.
- **Treat yourself right.** Take a relaxing bath or a long shower. Have your partner give you a massage. Wear clothing that comfortably fits and flatters your new pregnant shape. Let yourself know through your own actions that you are worthy and deserving of good things.
- **Express Yourself.** Keep a journal to record your journey through pregnancy, jotting down all the ordinary and extraor-dinary moments leading to the birth of your child. What will soon be precious memories is also a lasting testimony to your body's own strength and power.

Most important, feel good about yourself by making a commit-ment to a healthy pregnancy lifestyle. Go to all your prenatal care appointments, learn all you can about pregnancy and childbirth, eat nutrient-rich foods, exercise, get plenty of rest, and take your prenatal vitamin. Create a positive self-image from knowing you are doing everything in your power to achieve a healthy, happy plus-size pregnancy.

For more tips on how to look good and feel great throughout pregnancy, see chapter 8, "Celebrating Your Pregnancy."

To the Sisters Trying to Conceive

Reaching a Healthy—and Sane— Preconception Weight

How much should you weigh before becoming pregnant? Pregnancy books often advise readers to reach an "ideal weight" before conceiving. There is usually no explanation or guidance offered for what this ideal weight should be. Is ideal what you weighed in high school or on your wedding day? Is ideal synonymous with "when you were at your skinniest"? What these books don't understand is that, in our society, "ideal weight" and "fantasy weight" mean almost the same thing. For most women, ideal weight has become an unrealistic and unattainable goal; a number to think about for sheer self-torture.

If you are reading this before becoming pregnant, we advise you to focus your preconception efforts on reaching a healthy, sane weight for your body type and personal health history. To calculate what this actual number should be, take into consideration the following factors:

- **Know your BMI.** Medical experts agree that plus-size women who enter pregnancy with a BMI of 30 or higher are at greater risk of experiencing complications such as gestational diabetes, gestational hypertension, preeclampsia, and delivery by cesarean section. Reducing your BMI below 30 can reduce your risk for many of these complications. Take this into account when formulating any weight-loss goals. Other studies suggest that, no matter how many points you are above a normal BMI, losing even 10 percent of your body weight before conceiving may cut your odds for encountering complications.
- **Evaluate your health history.** Not only important once you become pregnant, your personal health history is an instructive preconception tool. Do you have high blood pressure? Do

you have diabetes? Is there a family history of diabetes and/or hypertension? Did you experience difficulties in a previous pregnancy? Answering yes to any of these questions indicates a BMI below 30 will almost certainly help you achieve a healthier pregnancy.

- **Evaluate your fertility.** As we will discuss in the next chapter, plus-size women who encounter ovulation problems are often able to restore their fertility by achieving a relatively small weight loss.
- **Talk to your doctor.** Make a preconception appointment with your OB or midwife to check out your general health and discuss a good weight for you to reach before trying to conceive. Your care provider can make a precise suggestion and if needed, refer you to a nutritionist to help you construct a sensible and practical preconception weight-loss strategy.

Whatever number you come up with—maybe it's the same as what you weigh right now, maybe it is a weight loss of 20, 30, 40, or more pounds—take good care of yourself as you prepare for conception. This means no crash dieting to quickly lose the weight. Starvation frequently results in severe vitamin and mineral deficiencies, meaning that losing weight through crash dieting can potentially do your pregnancy more harm than good. Your best bet is to eat a sensible diet and make sure to take a prenatal vitamin containing at least 400 micrograms (mcg) of folic acid every day.

2

FERTILITY
and WEIGHT

Getting Pregnant

During the months we were trying to conceive, I was so in tune with my body I swear I could feel myself ovulate. My husband called me the "fertility goddess."

—ANNA, age 26

YOUR ABILITY TO conceive relies on many factors: age, heredity, stress, correctly timing intercourse, preexisting medical conditions, quality and quantity of sperm provided by your partner, and yes, your weight. Are plus-size women more likely to have fertility problems? If you are reading this book, pregnant after only trying for one month (or not consciously trying at all), then your likely response to this question is *absolutely not!* For those of you who tried for months and years before conceiving, or are still trying, we know your answers are very different.

The first stop on the pregnancy journey, this chapter is devoted to how you ended up where you are right now. How *does* body weight affect fertility? We provide an in-depth look at fertility in plus-size women, including detailed information about fertility problems and polycystic ovary syndrome (PCOS), a common health concern among plus-size women. Reading this book before becoming pregnant? You will find sensible strategies to help you prepare for conception and enhance your fertility.

Fertility and Weight

FERTILITY AND WEIGHT are closely—and complexly—connected. You *do* need fat to be fertile (about 20 percent of your total body weight). Fat enables your body to carry out the staggering number of hormonal changes that must occur each month for ovulation, the release of an egg from one of your ovaries, to occur. Too much fat, however, can upset the body's delicate hormonal balance and disrupt normal ovulation. Irregular ovulation and/or lack of ovulation are two leading causes of fertility problems among plus-size women. Taking a closer look at your monthly cycle can help you see how the intricate relationship between your hormones, your weight, and your fertility really works.

Your Monthly Cycle and Your Weight: It's All about Balance

A new monthly cycle begins the day your period arrives. As soon as you begin menstruating, your body quickly begins preparing for another round of ovulation and another chance at becoming pregnant. Priming an egg for release requires the assistance of some powerful hormones. Your brain's pituitary gland increases the amount of certain hormones circulating in your bloodstream. One of these hormones, called FSH (follicle stimulating hormone) makes its way to your ovaries, helping a handful of eggs (from the hundreds of thousands contained in your ovaries) to ripen and mature. Eggs are contained in follicles, tiny fluid-filled cysts in the ovary. As eggs mature, one follicle (and sometimes two) grows larger than the others. This "dominant follicle" contains the lucky egg that will be released—just as soon as a few more hormonal changes take place.

Estrogen is another hormone hard at work during the first few weeks of your monthly cycle. Increasing amounts of estrogen trigger the lining of your uterus to thicken, readying it for the possibility that the egg about to be released will become fertilized and you will become pregnant. Rising estrogen levels also prompt a brief surge in LH (luteinizing hormone). This sudden hormonal spike causes the dominant follicle to rupture. Ovulation, the egg's discharge from the ruptured follicle, normally occurs two weeks before your next menstrual period begins (some women may feel a slight pinching pain during ovulation). If sperm are present as the recently freed egg enters the fallopian tube, conception may take place.

Without knowing if the released egg was fertilized, your body hedges its bets and keeps preparing for pregnancy. Estrogen, along with other hormones produced during ovulation, continue to rise and your uterine lining continues to thicken. If a fertilized egg does not arrive and implant in the uterus within two weeks, your body recognizes that conception did not take place. Hormone levels rapidly drop, your uterus sheds its thickened lining (menstruation), and the entire cycle begins again.

Plus-size women *may* produce higher-than-normal levels of estrogen. Remember, when it comes to hormones, it's all about balance. If there is too much estrogen already in your body as your monthly cycle begins, the amount of FSH released by your brain decreases. Lower-than-normal amounts of FSH might mean your eggs do not ripen and mature on schedule. If you are trying to conceive, irregularity in when you ovulate can seriously hamper your efforts. A hormonal imbalance could also result in the release of no egg at all. While all women occasionally have this type of cycle (called an anovulatory cycle), frequently missing out on ovulation results in fertility problems.

One Size Fits All?

So, IF YOU are pregnant right now, are you just lucky? Our discussion of fertility and weight is an excellent place to stress that any issue related to plus-size pregnancy is *never* "one size fits all." Every woman's body is different, regardless of how much she weighs.

Medical researchers, however, have spent quite a bit of time studying ovulation problems and conception rates among plus-size women. Their findings suggest that as a woman's body mass index (BMI)* increases, so does the *possibility* she will experience weight-related fertility problems. This means a woman whose BMI is above 30 (classified as an "obese" BMI) is more likely to encounter ovulation and fertility difficulties than a woman whose BMI is between 25 and 29 (considered "overweight"). While it is still unclear, there appear to be many other contributing factors behind why certain plus-size women have difficulty conceiving. Sometimes problems are not at all weight-based, but related to one of the other factors affecting fertility listed at the beginning of this chapter. All experts agree on a simple fact: being plus-sized does not guarantee fertility problems.

---

*Knowing your BMI helps you better understand the medical issues related to plus-size pregnancy. If you have not already done so, calculate your BMI using the chart on page 10.

Fertility Solutions

Are You Ovulating?

When monthly efforts to conceive do not result in pregnancy, consult with your doctor to pinpoint your infertility's likely cause. Before you set off for the doctor's office, gathering together some important health information can help both you and your doctor better understand what is happening—and not happening—during your monthly cycle. Are you ovulating? You can help answer that question by taking the following steps:

- **Chart your cycles.** Record the length of your monthly cycles over the past few months. Most women think their cycles must last precisely 28 days to be considered normal. In reality, a normal cycle can last anywhere from 22 to 35 days. Cycles shorter than 22 days, or cycles that fluctuate in length from month to month, might indicate ovulation problems. Also note how many days your period lasted and whether there was unusually heavy or light flow.
- **Take your temperature.** Tracking you body temperature throughout your cycle can reveal important clues about ovulation. Most women experience a slight dip in temperature (a few tenths of a degree *below* normal) just before ovulation and a slight rise in body temperature (less than one degree *above* normal) after ovulation. This higher body temperature lasts until just before your period begins, or longer if you are pregnant. If no shift in body temperature is detected, chances are you are not ovulating.

  For accurate tracking, use your *basal body temperature*. This is your temperature first thing in the morning before you get out of bed and start moving around. Take your temperature using a regular digital thermometer or a "metabolic thermometer" designed to only pick up small changes in temperature (from 95° to 100°F). One caveat to this method of predicting ovulation—elevated morning temperatures could also be the result of illness or a restless night. Keep your thermometer, along with a pad and pencil to record results, in a convenient spot next to your bed.

- **Check your cervical mucus.** Cervical mucus, what you have doubtlessly seen before as a sometimes clear and sometimes whitish vaginal discharge, plays an important role in predicting ovulation. For most of your cycle, cervical mucus is sticky and opaque. This is "unfertile cervical mucus," and its role is to trap and prevent sperm from crossing the cervix into the uterus. The same hormones responsible for preparing an egg to ovulate create changes in this mucus. For about five days leading up to ovulation, the mucus becomes clear and slippery. This "fertile mucus" allows sperm easier transport through the reproductive tract. As we'll explain later, time is of the essence when a sperm is in search of an egg. You can easily check your cervical mucus each day. Seeing a change from white and sticky to clear and slippery (and then back to white and sticky) is a good indication you are ovulating.
- **Create a fertility health record.** List any illnesses, medical conditions, stressful life events, or significant changes in your body over the last several months. Do the same for your partner. For both of you, include information about your use of medications, herbs, alcohol, tobacco, and/or illicit drugs. If you have conceived before, provide details about that, too. Did you have an easy time getting pregnant? Have you ever had a miscarriage? Have you ever carried a pregnancy to term? While irregular ovulation is a leading cause of infertility in plus-size women, this information can help uncover other underlying reasons for your infertility, such as blocked fallopian tubes or problems with sperm quality and/or quantity.

Going to your appointment with so many facts already in hand may reduce the amount of time necessary to diagnose your fertility difficulties. Educating yourself about your body is an empowering process, allowing both you and your doctor to make the best decisions for your care. At your visit, expect your doctor to uncover even more information about your fertility by running blood tests to check hormone levels and performing an X-ray or ultrasound scan to evaluate your reproductive organs.

It is important to note that for many women, talking to their regular doctor or a fertility specialist about conception difficulties, especially weight-related fertility problems, can feel awkward or intimidating. It absolutely should not be. If you do not have a regular

OB-GYN or primary care physician (or just don't feel comfortable talking about these issues with the doctor you are currently seeing), please read chapter 3, "Guide to Prenatal Health Care," for practical advice about finding excellent medical care.

Small Losses, Big Gains

I visited my gynecologist to find out why I was having such a hard time getting pregnant. We discussed my cycle in great detail; he ran some tests and asked me questions about my general health. According to my gynecologist, irregular ovulation appeared to be the likely cause of my fertility problems. He told me the best way to fix the problem was to lose weight. As I envisioned myself back on the crash diets, back on the weight-loss roller coaster that was partially to blame for why I weighed close to 200 pounds, I felt sick. I was making a mental grocery list of the ingredients in the cabbage soup diet, when he told me exactly how much weight I should lose.

I was told that for my weight, a twenty-pound weight loss would probably work to regulate ovulation and make it easier for me to predict when I was fertile. Just twenty pounds. My gynecologist told me to spread out the weight loss over a three-month period—no crash diets! He also told me to take another three months to maintain the weight loss, take a prenatal vitamin, and then begin trying. I went to a weight-loss support group at the hospital and gradually lost the weight. When we started up our conception efforts again, I became pregnant within two months. About a year and a half after that first appointment, I was burping and changing my newborn daughter.

—YOLANDA, age 29

IF YOUR DIFFICULTY conceiving is likely caused by disrupted ovulation, the most common treatment is weight loss. As Yolanda found out, the amount of weight loss needed to jumpstart your fertility is surprisingly small. Losing even 5 to 10 percent of your total body weight is often enough to bring your hormones back into balance and restore ovulation. For example, if you weigh 200 pounds, you will need to lose somewhere between 15 and 20 pounds. Your doctor can determine the amount you should lose for the best chance to resume regular ovulation.

Because you are gearing up for conception, shed pounds by eating a nutritious and balanced weight-loss diet. Crash diets and fad diets, stressing very low calorie menu plans or just eating one food group, often lead to deficiencies in the key vitamins and minerals needed to sustain a healthy pregnancy. To speed up weight loss, add thirty minutes or more of physical activity to your daily schedule. Pick activities you actually like—walking, swimming, riding a bike, and aerobics are usually good bets. If you have not exercised regularly in the past, start slowly (walk for ten or fifteen minutes a few times a week). As your stamina improves, gradually increase the length and intensity of your workout. See chapter 6 for more exercise suggestions and guidelines.

Maintaining your weight loss for a few months before actively trying to conceive allows your body time to replenish nutrients depleted during any weight-loss regimen. Be sure to take a daily vitamin supplement containing at least 400 mcg of folic acid.

Other Ways to Regulate Ovulation

BASED ON ITS success rate for so many women, weight loss is often the first treatment recommended. However, other options are available to achieve fertility. Some women who experience missed or irregular ovulation may be prescribed the synthetic fertility drug, clomiphine citrate (known to many by its brand name, Clomid). Clomiphine citrate "tells" the brain to release more FSH and LH. When these hormones increase, ovulation returns. Another alternative is to receive daily hormone injections (a mix of FSH and LH) to balance out elevated estrogen levels and reestablish ovulation. Both methods—clomiphene and hormone injections—may stimulate the release of more than one egg, resulting in higher rates of multiple birth pregnancy.

Whatever route you and your doctor take to remedy your fertility, remember that no one method works for 100 percent of all women. It might be necessary to try several treatment options before achieving the result you want.

Polycystic Ovary Syndrome (PCOS)

SOMETIMES HORMONAL IMBALANCES and disrupted ovulation result from causes other than the ones we have described so far in this chapter. Women diagnosed with polycystic ovary syndrome (PCOS), a hormonal and metabolic disorder, endure their own unique set of fertility challenges. PCOS affects nearly 6 million women of childbearing age in the United States. Approximately half of all diagnosed cases belong to plus-size women.

Polycystic ovaries are enlarged ovaries studded with numerous small cysts. Cysts form if the ovary's "dominant follicle" is unable to properly grow and prepare for ovulation due to hormonal interference. Instead of rupturing during ovulation, the immature follicle remains intact and creates a cyst. Women with PCOS frequently experience irregular cycles (with or without ovulation) or may temporarily stop menstruating. Because normal ovulation may occur during some cycles, conception *is* possible, but can certainly become more difficult to orchestrate.

Causes and Symptoms

Although researchers are not sure what exactly triggers the hormonal imbalance leading to PCOS, the syndrome is linked with elevated levels of testosterone. While all women naturally produce testosterone, women with PCOS manufacture higher-than-normal amounts. Some clues you have PCOS are testosterone-related. Acne, excess facial or body hair, and thinning scalp hair may indicate an overabundance of this hormone. Anxiousness and moodiness may also signal a hormonal imbalance.

Other symptoms of PCOS are directly related to disrupted ovulation. When the dominant follicle does not mature, the body can act as though it is still in the build-up to ovulation phase. This can go on for weeks—or even months—causing delayed or absent menstruation. Evidence for PCOS includes: cycles lasting longer than 5 weeks; heavy, prolonged periods; and going more than 2 months without menstruating (not caused by pregnancy).

PCOS and Plus-Size Women: The Insulin Connection

Approximately half of all women with PCOS can be classified as obese, and many more are considered overweight. These statistics have prompted researchers to look for a connection between body weight and PCOS. According to their studies, almost 75 percent of plus-size women with PCOS also have increased insulin resistance. *Insulin* is the hormone responsible for controlling blood glucose levels (sugar in your blood generated from the foods you eat). Insulin escorts glucose molecules from your bloodstream into individual cells where the glucose is then used as energy. When you develop insulin resistance, cells "resist" the insulin and do not allow glucose to enter. Large quantities of insulin must be produced to overcome the resistance and drive glucose into cells. Insulin resistance is often a precursor to Type II diabetes because eventually the body may not be able to manufacture enough insulin to keep up with demand. High blood sugar levels (diabetes) develop as a result.

There is a potent relationship between PCOS and insulin resistance. Because insulin is such a powerful hormone, large quantities of it are strong enough to trigger production of other hormones, including testosterone. This insulin-testosterone link in some plus-size women is most likely what activates the hormonal imbalance leading to PCOS. Researchers still don't completely understand the complete genetic and environmental factors behind why these plus-size women are more prone to insulin resistance in the first place, but lowering insulin levels has been shown effective in managing PCOS.

PCOS and Fertility: The Good News

I had no idea what was wrong with me. I was twenty-five and had pimples like a thirteen-year-old. I loved my job and was happily married, but I often felt anxious and moody. And then my periods started getting really wacky. I'd go for a few months without menstruating, even though the countless home pregnancy tests I bought all told me I wasn't pregnant. When I finally went to my doctor to find out what was wrong, I was diagnosed with something called polycystic ovary syndrome. It was a relief to find out there was a name to describe what I was experiencing, but I was also scared. Could I do anything to get better? How would this affect my future plans to become pregnant?

—GINA, age 26

Great strides have been made in recent years to help women with PCOS return hormone levels to normal range, reduce symptoms, and restore healthy cycles. If you are already diagnosed with PCOS—or suspect you have the condition based on the symptoms we described above—discuss with your doctor your specific concerns. You and your doctor can tailor a treatment plan to fit your needs, relying on the following methods shown to successfully manage PCOS and boost fertility:

- **Sensible weight loss:** Losing even a small amount of total body weight (5 to 10 percent) is often enough to bring hormone levels back into balance, alleviate symptoms, and restart normal ovulation. In one study of women with PCOS and disrupted ovulation, 70 percent of research participants who lost

5 percent of their body weight became pregnant without any
further medical intervention.

- **Attention to diet:** Whether you are on a weight-loss diet or
  not, pay attention to the foods you eat. Stay away from "refined
  carbohydrates" such as candy, soda, cakes, snack foods, and
  white bread. Eliminate foods from your diet that contain added
  sugar (read food labels for such ingredients as sucrose, glucose,
  fructose, honey, and high-fructose corn syrup). These easily
  absorbed carbohydrates quickly enter the bloodstream and
  create a sudden spike in blood glucose. Your body responds by
  producing large amounts of insulin. As described above,
  higher-than-normal insulin levels spur the production of testosterone and set off the hormonal imbalance leading to PCOS.

  Opt for foods that will keep blood sugar levels on an even
  keel. For best results, create an eating plan centered around
  whole grains (brown rice, whole wheat bread, steel-cut oats),
  fruits, vegetables, and healthy sources of protein and fat. See
  chapter 5, "Prenatal Nutrition," for more information about
  incorporating whole grains into your diet.

- **Exercise:** Regular physical activity is a natural way to keep
  your body's hormones in balance. When you exercise, your cells
  become "hungry" for energy. Cells drop their resistance and
  more easily allow glucose (the cell's energy source) to enter. You
  do not need to produce large quantities of insulin as a result.
  Something as simple as briskly walking for twenty minutes
  after eating a meal helps prevent insulin levels from surging.

- **"Insulin sensitizers":** Certain drugs make your cells less
  resistant to insulin, allowing your body to produce decreased
  amounts of the hormone. Usually prescribed to Type II dia-
  betics for blood sugar control, insulin-sensitizing drugs (such
  as Metformin) also prove helpful to plus-size women with
  PCOS. Lower insulin levels mean excess testosterone production is not stimulated. Studies show PCOS-related symptoms frequently decrease (and fertility increases) in women
  who use an insulin-sensitizer.

- **Fertility drugs:** Women with PCOS may be prescribed
  clomiphine citrate or receive hormone injections to induce
  ovulation (usually a shot of FSH to properly mature the follicle and egg). Fertility drugs might be used in conjunction
  with any of the other methods mentioned above.

Maintaining a healthy lifestyle is important for all women with PCOS, whether they are preparing for conception or not. Women who take steps to balance their hormones often see their PCOS-related symptoms dramatically improve.

Enhance Your Fertility

YOU KNOW YOU are ready. You met with your doctor and got the thumbs up about your general health and weight. Your ovulation appears regular. You are taking a prenatal vitamin. You want to have a baby. And now the fun really begins, trying to conceive! The following are a few basic strategies and tips to help you and your partner improve your chances of getting pregnant:

- **Timing is everything.** You are most fertile during the five days surrounding ovulation. Hormonal changes preparing an egg for release prompt the cervix to become more sperm-friendly. Cervical mucus, normally sticky and difficult for sperm to move through, is now slippery and chemically altered to protect the sperm. The muscles of the cervix relax and the cervix becomes more open, enabling sperm to quickly advance into the uterus and fallopian tubes (some sperm will stay behind near the cervix and only approach the fallopian tube when the egg arrives). Sperm can live for up to five days in this environment.

  After ovulation, the egg leaves the ovary and enters the fallopian tube. The egg emits hormonal signals to announce its presence and entice sperm to approach. While sperm can remain active for several days in your reproductive tract, an egg is viable once it is in the fallopian tube for 24 to 48 hours. Fertilization must take place within this narrow timeframe.

  To give sperm the best chance of being in the right place at the right time, concentrate your baby-making efforts on these five most fertile days. Track your cycle to pinpoint likely ovulation. Check your cervical mucus to make sure conditions are favorable. Many experts agree that having sex every other day during your fertile time is more effective than daily intercourse. This is especially true for men with low sperm counts. How you choose to maximize your fertile period is up to you and your partner. Whatever you do, avoid making sex a chore.

- **Chill out.** Male testicles are suspended on the outside of the body to maintain the slightly cooler temperature needed for optimal sperm production (two degrees lower than the rest of the body). Regularly soaking in a hot bath, frequent hot tub use, or tight-fitting briefs can raise the temperature inside the scrotum. Frequent exposure to high temperatures can result in lower sperm production and a higher-than-normal percentage of abnormal sperm. The cure for this is simple. Rather than a hot soak, take a warm shower; opt for the swimming pool and not the hot tub; wear boxers instead of briefs. Experts report it can take up to two months for sperm production to recover from overexposure to high temperatures.

- **Beware of fertility health hazards.** If you or your partner use any type of medication or herbal supplement, check with your doctor to make sure what you are taking does not interfere with sperm production or ovulation. Certain ulcer, irritable bowel syndrome, and high blood pressure medications have a negative effect on sperm quality and/or quantity in men. For women, thyroid replacement therapy might create an imbalance of reproductive hormones and disrupt ovulation. Some experts believe such herbal supplements as St. John's wort, echinacea, and ginkgo biloba pose harm to sperm. Women should avoid blue cohosh, sold in herbal remedies for PMS. It is equally important to make sure your medications and herbal remedies are safe for fetal development once you do conceive. When in doubt, check it out!

    Other fertility health hazards both of you should avoid include: alcohol consumption (no alcohol for you, reduced drinking for your partner), smoking, recreational drug use, and exposure to pesticides and chemical toxins.

- **Deal with your emotions:** If you are like many women, months and months of trying unsuccessfully to become pregnant may lead to deep feelings of depression. According to researchers from the Harvard Behavioral Medicine Program for Infertility, dealing with your negative emotions may be the key to unlocking your fertility. In a joint study between Harvard and the National Institute of Mental Health, women who received intense emotional support, talking with other women in the same situation and learning relaxation techniques (like meditation), saw great improvement in their ability to conceive. Why? Powerful emotional distress, like depression, may trigger hormonal imbalances that disrupt ovulation. According to these researchers, feeling calmer, happier, and less stressed makes it easier to become pregnant.

To boost your chances of conceiving, try a yoga class to see if it helps you let go of stress and anxiety. Get in touch with others in your same situation by contacting your local chapter of RESOLVE, a national support group for women (and their partners) with fertility difficulties. And, of course, share your feelings with your doctor.

- **Enjoy sex.** Last but not least, find pleasure in your efforts to conceive. If sex during your fertile period is becoming robotic and not very satisfying, you may be missing out on your body's own natural fertility-enhancer: orgasm. The muscular contractions of a female orgasm create a suction effect between the cervix and the vagina allowing more sperm to pass quickly through the cervix—a head start on their race toward the egg.

The most common fertility tip from the big, beautiful, and pregnant sisterhood is simple: *be patient*. No matter how long it takes to get pregnant, enjoy the process of making a family (or making a family grow). While it might be nice to have a positive result after only a month, that's almost always the exception, not the rule. Relax and enjoy this special time of intimacy between you and your partner.

If you just read this section—or this chapter—and are amazed at the incredible number of conditions needed to start a pregnancy, keep reading. Remember, conception is only the first stop in your extraordinary nine-month journey.

3

THE SISTERHOOD'S GUIDE TO PRENATAL HEALTH CARE

Let Go of the Past

I ventured off to my first prenatal visit with the worst case of jitters ever experienced in my life. Questions crowded my racing thoughts. Would I receive the "weight lecture" from my doctor? Would I be told all the horrible things destined to happen to my plus-size pregnancy? Could I hope, at least a little, to be treated with dignity and respect? I opened the office door and took a deep breath, bracing for whatever came my way.

—STACEY, age 23

WHAT IS IT about going to the doctor that makes so many plus-size women so uncomfortable? Maybe it's anxiety about the inevitable weigh-in or those ill-fitting paper gowns that never seem to cover what they should. Perhaps it's encountering physicians who lecture about proper diet and exercise in tones suggesting plus-size women sit on the couch all day eating potato chips, or the fumbling excuses some sisters feel compelled to make for how the extra weight got there in the first place.

Whatever might hamper your ability to feel completely at ease with members of the medical community is no longer acceptable now that you are pregnant. Prenatal care monitors your overall health and provides important information about your baby's growth and development. As a plus-size woman, your capacity to trust, confide in, and question your prenatal care provider is critical. You need to feel confident that all your concerns will be addressed with honesty and dignity. There is no room for fear, shame, and guilt when it comes to making sure your pregnancy is a healthy success.

This chapter arms you with the information you need to establish and maintain an open and assertive relationship with your prenatal healthcare provider, whether it is an obstetrician, family practitioner, or midwife. We'll show you steps to locating a supportive and size-friendly provider, how to make the most of your first visit, why common appointment tests and routines are so important, and what to do if your provider just doesn't work out. Most importantly, you will acquire all the tools necessary to receive the excellence in care you have always deserved.

Finding Supportive, Size-Friendly Prenatal Care

During my first prenatal checkup, the midwife asked right off the bat if I had questions or concerns. We chatted a bit about general issues and, when I felt comfortable, I mentioned how I was worried about what could happen because I was overweight and pregnant. She politely responded to my fears, carefully stressing that being overweight did not automatically mean that I would develop a complication, but it might entail monitoring my pregnancy more closely. We discussed weight gain goals and a safe exercise plan. At the end of the visit, she had information readily available for me to take home and read.

Every time I saw my provider, she complimented me on my steady but controlled weight gain and wanted to know what I was doing to enjoy my pregnancy. Because we had spoken so honestly and openly at the first visit, it was easy for me to be up front about whatever was on my mind. I remember the needless worry and anxiety I put myself through before my first appointment with her. At five foot six and two hundred and forty pounds I thought my provider would constantly criticize me. Nothing could be further from the truth. I had a beautiful and healthy pregnancy, and a beautiful and healthy baby. My birthing experience was more enjoyable than I had anticipated because I trusted this person to provide me with the best of care.

—LISA, age 30

IF YOU ARE not completely comfortable with the OB-GYN you see for annual appointments or have never had a regular provider, you will need to search for an obstetrician, midwife, or family practitioner to care for you during your pregnancy.

Prenatal providers who win the sisterhood's approval treat plus-size women with the same respect accorded all their patients. "Size-friendly" providers take time to listen to their patients' questions and are considerate yet honest in their answers. In their care, pregnant plus-size women are free from any guilt or shame over not having lost weight before conceiving. If anything, you will receive a little more TLC than the average patient because size-friendly providers understand the issues plus-size women face and know that a member of the sisterhood might need added emotional support.

Because it is next to impossible to tell which prenatal care provider from the dozens listed in the yellow pages will best care for a plus-size pregnancy, here are some strategies to help you strike obstetric gold:

- **Ask other women for advice.** Finding out the good, bad, and the ugly about prenatal care providers in your area can save you a lot of stress and misery. Members of the sisterhood who work with you, are in your church and community groups, and count themselves among your close friends and family, can give you the skinny on how different care providers treat over-weight women. Start making a list of these referrals.

  Survey the childbearing women in your immediate vicinity, even if they are thin. Medical professionals who are truly car-ing and supportive don't discriminate on the basis of patient size. So, when your lanky cousin raves about how great her OB is, take that name into consideration, too.

- **Ask your current doctor.** If your primary care or family physician is to your liking, trust his or her judgment and ask for referrals. Ask specifically for names of obstetricians whom your doctor thinks provide the best care for larger women.

- **Check with the hospital's referral service.** Some hospitals have consultants on hand who match obstetricians and other specialists with your personal preferences. It's almost like a doctor-patient dating service. Some sisters have found won-derful size-friendly providers this way but, just like bad blind dates, a few OBs who were promised to have "great personal-ities" turned out to be total duds.

- **Attend a "Meet the Doctors" night.** Large practices or doc-tors who belong to a call group hold these events every few weeks or months. Each doctor usually presents a mini-lecture to the audience on some aspect of labor and delivery with time at the end for questions and answers. In addition to a basic childbirth overview, these gatherings are a chance for women and their partners to get to know—or at least recognize the face of—the many possible doctors who might be present in the delivery room. Maybe some provider's style and personality will strike you as the perfect match. At the very least, you will leave more informed about what will happen to you in nine short months! Call some offices in the phone book and ask about the next presentation date.

To narrow down your list of prospective prenatal care providers, take into account some practical considerations and personal preferences to help you make your final choice:

- **Contact your insurance company.** Delete from the list any providers not covered by your insurance plan.
- **Large or small practice?** There are advantages and disadvantages to each practice size. Multi-obstetrician offices, some with a dozen doctors or more, will often be able to perform blood work, ultrasounds, and other obstetric testing on site rather than sending you to the hospital. Extended hours and an in-house pharmacy may also be available. Be prepared, however, for practice policy to vary when it comes to how often you see your chosen obstetrician. Some practices alternate between a nurse practitioner and OB for the first few visits. Others require patients to rotate appointments through all the practice's obstetricians until the latter months of pregnancy.

    Before you decide on an OB in a large practice, inquire about the visit schedule. Some offices are very rigid about rotating appointments, but many accept requests to schedule all visits with the same provider. Be sure to ask around for opinions on the other obstetricians in the practice. Unfortunately, a few sisters report encountering obstetricians during these rotating appointments who have no business caring for overweight women.

    Solo or small practices may offer you a greater chance to bond with your prenatal care team during pregnancy. While you will most likely need to go to the hospital lab for all but the most routine tests, it can be comforting to see the same doctor (probably even the same nurse and receptionist) at every visit. If you decide on a solo or small practice, make sure to find out if your obstetrician is part of a call group, a number of doctors who agree to cover delivery shifts at the hospital. Most obstetricians will offer opportunities for you to briefly meet the other doctors before the big day (see "Meet the Doctors" above), but it can still be a bit disconcerting to find that the person on the receiving end of the delivery table is little more than a complete stranger.

- **Visit area hospitals.** Tour the birthing wings at the hospitals where the doctors on your list are affiliated. If you are having a hard time choosing between two highly recommended providers, actually seeing the place where you will give birth might be a deciding factor in your choice. You can find out a provider's designated hospital from your insurance company or by calling their office (also call the hospital to see if an appointment is needed to visit). Some hospitals have gone out of their way to cultivate a pleasant, homey atmosphere by installing natural wood floors and soft lighting, hanging pretty wallpaper, and providing a fold-out bed for your partner. You might find that there are whirlpool baths at your disposal or an entire water-birthing suite.

   Once your baby is born, see if the maternity wing allows for "rooming in," or keeping your baby with you for the duration of your stay if no medical intervention is required. On a more practical note, some women find it important that the hospital have a NICU (neonatal intensive care unit) in the event more serious medical care is needed.

- **Interview your top choices.** Call a few of the names on your list and make an appointment just to chat. In your conversation with these prospective care providers, be open and honest about how you want to be treated. Ask about their attitudes toward plus-size women and how experienced they are with caring for overweight pregnancies. Allow them to do a lot of the talking, and listen carefully to get a handle on their personality and style. Be forewarned that some providers are more willing than others to schedule "chat time" (this policy may be telling in itself). Although no examination is taking place, be prepared to pay the standard appointment rate.

- **Change can be a good thing.** Nearly 1 in 5 women changes doctors due to dissatisfaction with care. So if your top choice turns out to be the wrong choice, take comfort in knowing that you are not alone in moving on. If you have to make a switch,

submitted and then asked me if I had any questions. Any nervousness that had dissipated thus far came back at full force. Almost as though it were someone else talking I heard my own voice start to say, "I'm concerned about my weight . . ."

Thirty minutes later I sat in my car, clutching my pamphlets of prenatal health information, replaying over and over again the answer just given to me by the obstetrician. It certainly was not what I, in my anxiousness and pessimism, had expected. Her response had actually been positive. In a respectful and nonjudgmental way, the doctor calmly explained that being overweight might make me at higher risk for certain pregnancy complications, but in absolutely no way doomed me to them. She reassured me that given my pretty low-risk health history, it was highly likely that I would be among the vast majority of larger women who have healthy pregnancies, healthy deliveries, and healthy babies.

—SUZIE, age 35

Especially if this is your first pregnancy, first time meeting your prenatal care provider, or first attempt at being up front with a medical professional about your weight, don't worry if the initial prenatal visit is preceded by bouts of anxiety. We offer the following tips and advice to help reduce first appointment nervousness and help you begin your relationship with your provider in as relaxed and confident a manner as possible:

- **Get organized!** Buy a notebook so you can record your prenatal health information. Use this notebook throughout your pregnancy to write down questions, future appointment times and test dates, phone numbers, and hospital information.
- **Learn the lingo.** Introduce yourself to the new lingo you will be hearing (for example, Braxton-Hicks, fundus, placenta) by browsing a few pregnancy Web sites.
- **Take the day off from work.** You want to be as relaxed as possible for this appointment.
- **Decide if anyone should accompany you.** Some women have their partners with them at every appointment, whereas others prefer sharing postvisit instant replays. Will having your mom or best friend there help you to feel more confident? Then bring her along. Most care providers will completely welcome your support person.

What Should I Ask? What Should I Say?

Take time before the appointment to jot down your concerns in your notebook. Before heading out, edit the questions into one coherent list, leaving room in between to write in the answers.

WEIGHT-RELATED QUESTIONS:
- What experience do you have working with overweight women?
- What impact will my weight have on my pregnancy?
- What should my weight gain be month by month?
- Do I need a special diet?
- What are some good low impact prenatal exercises?
- Where can I go to find out more information about being overweight and pregnant?

GENERAL CONCERNS:
- Whom do I call in case of an emergency?
- What kinds of tests can I expect?
- Do you only share test results if there is cause for concern?
- What kinds of childbirth preparation classes are offered?
- Can you recommend some strategies to deal with morning sickness, varicose veins, backache, etc.?

Weightier Issues

If you have never openly discussed your weight with a medical professional before, sharing with your provider the concerns you have about being overweight and pregnant can be a frightening experience. Admitting you fear receiving substandard treatment due to size may be intimidating. Take a deep breath and stay focused on the big picture— that you want this pregnancy and your baby to be as healthy as possible. Never forget how plentiful the rewards are for taking a risk and being honest and direct with your prenatal care provider.

Hearing reasonable explanations of what plus-size women might encounter during pregnancy can replace troublesome thoughts with real information, helping you to make more informed choices. Asking your provider at the very first meeting if he/she is comfortable treating an overweight woman might feel awkward. If the answer is not what you want to hear, be glad you only wasted one appointment determining that this person is not the right care provider for you. Most importantly, taking charge and being the first to address your weight boosts your confidence and allows you to set the tone for how you want to be treated.

Beyond Talking: Appointment Routines

ONCE THE NERVOUSNESS of the first appointment is over, your prenatal care should settle into a predictable rhythm. In addition to provider "talk-time," most standard visits include several simple procedures, with each designed to measure the health and well-being of your pregnancy. Becoming an empowered health-care consumer means understanding these many tests and routines.

Weigh-In

Even if you see the doctor's scale as some sort of personal nemesis, it provides important information about your baby's physical growth and your health. You are weighed at each appointment. If you gain too much or too little weight from visit to visit, your doctor may look at this as a red flag that something else is going on, including: a very large or small baby, too much or too little amniotic fluid, or preeclampsia (if rapid weight gain is accompanied by high blood pressure and protein in the urine).

Depending on your prepregnancy weight, your provider will recommend a general weight-gain goal. Discuss with your individual provider what is best for you, but, as described in chapter 1, plus-size women should generally gain between 15 and 25 pounds total during pregnancy. This breaks down to about 3 to 4 pounds per month during the second and third trimesters.

This limited weight gain does not leave much room for error when you step on the scale. Monitoring little details like clothing choice can ensure a more accurate weight measurement. Wear the same types of clothes to each appointment and check to make sure something like your cell phone isn't bogging you down. Pay attention to your shoes! If you wore them during the first appointment's weigh-in, wear shoes whenever you step on the scale. Some shoes can throw off measurements by a few pounds. Try to make appointments at the same time during the day. Weight can fluctuate throughout the day as much as 5 pounds.

Another scale issue some sisters deal with is the weight announcement—223! 305! 167! Doctor's office scales are usually in the hallway, a location that is anything but private. Having your measurement proclaimed to anyone within earshot may be embarrassing and more than a bit disconcerting. Even if no one else is around, some women just don't like hearing the number spoken aloud. Tell the person who performs the weigh-in (if it is the same person each time; if not, speak directly with your provider) that instead of announcing your weight measurement, you simply want like to hear the number of pounds gained or lost since the last visit.

If you weigh over 350 pounds, the measurement limit on most standard doctor's scales, your provider's office should have an attachment that converts a standard scale to one that will accommodate higher weights. If this is a concern for you, call the office to verify that they have the attachments and know how to use them.

Urine Check

A urine sample is taken at the beginning of each visit. For the first visit you may need to drink a little extra water, but don't worry, pretty soon you will be peeing on demand. The nurse or physician's assistant immediately tests your urine for protein and sugar. If you have developed gestational diabetes, a condition in which your body becomes temporarily resistant to the effects of insulin and cannot properly metabolize all the carbohydrates (sugars) you eat, extra sugar may get dumped into your urine. Excess protein in the urine, when accompanied by high blood pressure, may indicate preeclampsia, a condition in which blood vessels become constricted and oxygen flow to the fetus may become impaired. Protein in the urine may also indicate a urinary tract infection.

Blood Pressure

Blood pressure is how much force blood exerts against the walls of your arteries. Your blood stream carries oxygen and other vital nutrients to your growing baby. When blood pressure is significantly higher than normal (more than 140/90), blood vessels are constricted and the amount of nourishment your baby receives may be diminished. Severely constricted blood flow may result in a low-birth-weight baby. Because blood pressure is such an important indicator of your pregnancy's overall health, blood pressure is measured at every prenatal visit.

Blood pressure measurements are given in two numbers: the amount of pressure in the arteries as the heart contracts (systolic pressure) and pressure in the arteries when the heart rests between beats (diastolic pressure). A normal blood pressure reading is 120 (systolic)/80 (diastolic). If your blood pressure has been normal and then measures above 140/90, you will be diagnosed with gestational hypertension, a pregnancy-associated form of high blood pressure. If high blood pressure is accompanied by protein in the urine, it indicates the more serious complication, preeclampsia.

Make sure your blood pressure readings are as accurate as possible. If you did not have high blood pressure before becoming pregnant and your readings begin to creep above 120/80, evaluate when and who is taking your blood pressure. While elevated readings could indeed mean that you are developing gestational hypertension, "white-coat hypertension," the spiking of blood pressure due to nervousness, is a very real phenomenon for some women. Blood pressure readings are usually taken by a nurse or physician's assistant at the beginning of your appointment. If you feel anxiety from the time you enter the office until you finally see your OB and get the thumbs-up that all is well, taking your blood pressure as soon as you walk in might yield a stress-induced measurement, and not your true reading. Feeling uncomfortable with the person doing the squeezing can also produce high measurements.

If you think white-coat hypertension is an issue for you, try some breathing and relaxation exercises before you enter the office. If this does not work, talk to your provider and request that someone with whom you feel comfortable takes your blood pressure, or that the reading be taken toward the end of the appointment when you are more relaxed.

Blood pressure readings in plus-size women may also be thrown off due to an improperly fitting cuff. Larger women require larger cuffs in order to receive accurate measurements. Studies have shown that using a too-small blood pressure cuff can produce falsely high readings. Some plus-women may actually have normal blood pressure, but a cuff that is too small makes the measurement appear higher than normal. Bring up cuff size with your OB, if you think this may be an issue. Your arm can be easily measured to determine whether a larger cuff would fit your needs.

Please see chapter 4, "Trimester by Trimester: Your Medical Concerns Addressed," for further information about blood pressure, gestational hypertension, and preeclampsia.

Fundal Height

Your prenatal care provider relies on fundal height measurements to determine if your baby is growing properly. To find the fundal height, a tape measure is run from the pubic bone, near where the uterus starts, to the fundus, the name given to the uppermost part of your ever-expanding uterus. Between weeks 20 and 34, the number of centimeters between these two points roughly corresponds to the age in weeks of your baby. In other words, a fundal height of 29 cm corresponds to a fetus that is 29 weeks old. Since this measurement is taken at each appointment, an unusual jump of a few centimeters or no growth between visits may cause your provider to order an ultrasound to make sure baby's development is on track.

In order to get the most accurate fundal height possible, the tape measure must be placed directly on the skin. You don't need to undress for this, just lift up your shirt and push down your pants to reveal your belly. Your provider then palpates the uterus, meaning he/she will press down on your skin until the pubic bone and fundus are felt. In later pregnancy, pressing down on the pubic bone may cause varying degrees of discomfort.

If you carried extra weight in the stomach area prepregnancy, obtaining an accurate fundal height measurement might be a bit tricky. The additional flesh becomes part of the measurement and can add a few centimeters. Discrepancies between fundal height and gestational age may also relate to your baby's position (breech/transverse or headfirst), amniotic fluid levels, and position of the baby's head in relation to the pelvis.

Your provider should demonstrate patience if a little extra time is needed for a proper measurement or politely explain why the fundal height might not be a reliable source of information in your situation. If it is too difficult to get an accurate fundal height measurement, you will most likely undergo a few additional ultrasounds to check your baby's growth rate. One sister found herself in this predicament when, at 30 weeks, her uterus measured 40 cm! She was quickly scheduled for a follow-up ultrasound and was relieved when the monitor showed a healthy baby right on target for 30 weeks' gestational development.

Fetal Heart Doppler

Another way your baby's well being is evaluated at each visit, starting around the third month, is to measure the fetal heart rate. Sliding a fetal heart Doppler instrument across your belly until baby's heartbeat is heard, your provider checks to make sure the heart is beating within a certain range, usually 110 to 160 beats per minute.

Carrying extra weight in the stomach area prepregnancy might affect how easy it is to find your baby's heartbeat (think soundproofed room). As when measuring fundal height, your provider has no reason to be anything but helpful and calm during this procedure. With a bit of persistence and a little patience, chances are the heartbeat will be heard loud and clear. Realize, too, that sometimes it's not extra girth that is the problem. Inside every pregnant woman is a little acrobat who—until pregnancy's latter months—has plenty of room to hide!

Once your provider locates your baby's heartbeat, don't leave subsequent visits without hearing it. Your provider should never shrug this off with the "too-much-padding-we'll-try-again-next-time" excuse. If needed, a basic ultrasound to check heart rate can be performed—often right in the office.

Recognizing and Dealing with Inadequate Care

My doctor never once mentioned my weight. I never brought it up, either. At five foot four and two hundred twenty pounds, I felt incredibly fat and I worried constantly about the health of my pregnancy. I was too embarrassed to bring up these fears with my doctor.

I gave birth to a healthy, beautiful baby boy who weighed less than expected, six pounds five ounces. Part of me was grateful my doctor never gave me a hard time (I had heard horror stories about that) but I was disappointed that so much of my pregnancy was spent worrying and feeling bad.

To this day, I wonder why my doctor never brought up my weight. During visits, I felt like my weight issue was the pink elephant in the room we both chose to ignore. She seemed to be all business, very few "how are you feeling" kinds of questions. Although I was torn up about what my weight might do to my baby, it was a relief not to have to ask or answer any uncomfortable questions. She seemed to have very little interest in me personally and that suited me just fine at the time. Looking back, I wish I had spoken up about my concerns.

—ANNIE, age 34

THE SEARCH FOR good prenatal care can sometimes seem like the modern day version of a familiar fairy tale. Some providers are too critical and fulfill the sisterhood's worst nightmares of biased, inferior treatment. Some providers, like Annie's, are too aloof and never take a real interest in their patients as individual women. They fail to understand that members of the sisterhood may need a little extra encouragement or time to ask weight-related questions. Other providers are "just right" and intuitively understand how to help plus-size women achieve healthy and happy pregnancies.

Although many women obtain a happily-ever-after relationship with their provider on the first try, what's a sister to do when faced with unsatisfactory prenatal care? While it might seem easy to simply pick up the phone and make an appointment with another practice, consider the following suggestions for dealing with a disappointing provider:

- **Speak up!** One sister reported that, at almost every visit her doctor made some remark about how he could not believe how good her blood pressure readings were. "It was the incredulous tone that got to me," Yvonne recounted. "What I really heard was, 'Wow, I thought all you fat women had high blood pressure. You're really lucky.' When I finally confronted my doctor about this annoying habit, he apologized profusely and told me he had no idea it sounded like that, but he could definitely see my point. He smoothed over the whole situation with some self-deprecating humor and everything was fine. I'm glad I spoke up instead of gritting my teeth through the rest of my appointments with him."

  If your provider says or implies something that upsets you, bring it to his or her attention. Politely confront your provider about unwelcome or confusing comments. A simple, "excuse me?" from a patient is usually enough to make a provider stop and rethink or rephrase his/her comments. Write your provider a letter to express what's bothering you, if voicing your concerns on paper makes you more comfortable. Many patient-provider issues are easily resolved with better communication. If you are not satisfied with how your concerns are addressed, you will need to decide whether or not it's time to find a new provider.

- **Make a change.** If you feel that appointments are rushed and you never have enough time to ask questions, stress that you have some issues you need to discuss. Instead of holding off on your questions until the end of the visit, begin with them. Be open and hold nothing back. Carefully observe how your provider responds. Maybe he/she was just innocently clueless and your initiative jump-starts his/her ability to compassionately address your concerns.

  Rushed visits may have other causes. Do you always schedule visits at 4:45 p.m. on a Friday? Does the practice have a policy of double-booking appointments? Request an additional visit just for talk-time, and schedule prenatal appointments early in the morning before the daily backlog begins. If, despite your best efforts, you spend more time finding a parking spot than talking with your provider, it's probably a good idea to consider a change.

- **Get a second opinion.** One sister confided that, after listening to her provider's exaggerated sighs when extra time was needed to find the fetal heartbeat, she hung on for one more visit to see if her provider's attitude would finally improve. When the nurse took her vitals, the sister asked why the doctor always seemed so irritated during visits. The nurse's reaction made it very clear that she no more liked working for this doctor than this sister liked being that doctor's patient! The second opinion from this candid nurse confirmed her instinct that this provider was not the one for her.

If you do change providers, let the old provider know, through a letter or a phone call, the reasons why you left. Be honest, stating factual examples of how the person fell short of your expectations, and clarifying what your expectations were, such as, "During each of my last three visits, you saw me for barely more than five minutes, and brushed aside my questions. I need a doctor who will take the time to listen to my concerns." It will be an emotionally cleansing release for you, and may be a sorely needed wake-up call for this particular provider. On a more practical note, request your medical records be sent to the new practice ASAP. It helps if a new provider is able to review your prenatal health history before your first meeting.

When it comes to receiving excellent prenatal care, never forget a simple truth. Successfully caring for a plus-size pregnancy demands more than just a medical degree. It requires an attitude that every woman, regardless of her size, is entitled to compassion and support throughout her pregnancy.

4

TRIMESTER *by* TRIMESTER:
Your Medical Concerns Addressed

Important Questions

Will I have a successful pregnancy? Is my baby healthy? What exactly is happening to my body? These commonly asked pregnancy questions are especially on your mind as a plus-size mom-to-be. You most likely have other, more weight-related concerns: *Should I lose weight now that I'm pregnant? Why am I being asked to have so many ultrasounds? Is a plus-size pregnancy automatically considered high risk? Will my baby have a high birth weight?*

This chapter provides you with direct and balanced answers to all your most pressing pregnancy questions. Divided into the three trimesters, each section begins with a brief summary of your baby's development and what changes to expect in your body. As you read this chapter, jot down any questions you have (whether they are the same ones reported here, or different) and ask them of your own provider. While our answers are based on current research and Dr. van der Ziel's extensive experience caring for plus-size women and their pregnancies, your provider knows best how certain medical issues might impact your pregnancy.

First Trimester (Weeks 1–13)

Your Baby: Beginnings

THE FIRST STEP to any pregnancy is, of course, conception. When a sperm fertilizes an egg, the two unite to form a single cell. Inside this tiny speck is all the complex information needed to create a human being. Conception usually takes place in one of the fallopian tubes, unless you conceive through in vitro fertilization (IVF) or another technologically assisted method.

The single cell does not wait long to begin its nine-month transformation. The fertilized egg rapidly undergoes cell division as it travels down the fallopian tube into the uterus, a distance of about 3¼ inches. Now called a *blastocyst*, the fertilized egg resembles a hollow ball of cells. The blastocyst embeds itself into the soft lining of your uterus in a process known as *implantation*. This entire process, from conception to implantation, takes about seven days.

Each cell created from the fertilized egg has a specific mission. Once implantation is successful, the cells attached to the uterine wall begin to form the *placenta*, the organ responsible for providing your baby with nourishment throughout pregnancy. Other cells develop into the *umbilical cord*, the pipeline between the placenta and your baby, as well as the amniotic sac, the fluid-filled membrane that provides baby with a cushion of protection until delivery.

And what about that baby? Last but not least, a specialized group of cells rapidly produce the main attraction. Over the next few weeks intense development takes place. The body's organ systems (nervous system, digestive system, circulatory system, etc.) quickly form and, by about eight weeks after conception, all are in place. They will develop and mature as the months progress.

A NOTE ABOUT DATING: Your pregnancy is dated from the first day of your last menstrual period (LMP). This is sometimes called your pregnancy's "menstrual age" or your baby's "gestational age." Fertilization probably took place 2 weeks (14 days) after the first day of your LMP. Why and how this is used is further explained in the Q&A section.

Milestones

MONTHS ONE AND TWO (WEEKS 1–8)
- The brain and spine develop four weeks after your LMP, right around the time you first notice a missed period.
- Your baby, now called an *embryo,* has a beating heart by week 5.
- Arms and leg buds appear, with fingers and toes visible by week 6
- Lungs, ears, eyes, and all other essential organs begin to form by week 8.

MONTH THREE (WEEKS 9–13)
- Officially called a *fetus* as the third month begins, your baby will grow to approximately three inches in the next few weeks.
- Your baby's face is well formed. Eyelids develop and stay closed until the end of the second trimester.
- Limbs (arms and legs) are long and thin. The fetal head is disproportionately larger than the rest of your baby's body. This will change during the second trimester.
- The fetus spontaneously moves about your uterus, although you are unable to detect this early activity. Your baby is now strong enough to make a fist.

Your Body: Getting into the Pregnancy Groove

As your baby transforms from a cluster of cells into a full-fledged fetus, your body must adapt to being pregnant. Pregnancy hormones, released soon after conception, send out signals that extra work is needed to nourish your baby and prepare for childbirth. This surge of hormones is necessary, but carries with it some unwelcome side effects. Fatigue, increased urination, morning sickness (nausea and/or vomiting) and food aversions are all typical first trimester inconveniences.

Emotionally, you might be noticeably more moody, sometimes feeling exhilarated one minute and anxious the next. Because pregnancy symptoms vary so widely among women, it's hard to predict which specific physical and emotional characteristics your pregnancy will include. Every woman, of every size, adjusts to pregnancy in her own unique way. Any symptoms you do encounter usually diminish or completely disappear (thankfully) as the first trimester draws to a close.

Common Experiences

MONTHS ONE AND TWO (WEEKS 1–8)

- In the earliest weeks of pregnancy, many women experience breast tingling and tenderness. These are often the first signs of pregnancy, even before a missed period is noticed.
- Blood vessels, especially on the breasts and abdomen, may become more pronounced. The amount of blood in your body increases to bring nourishment to your growing baby. Your total blood volume increases by about 15 percent during the first trimester alone. By the end of pregnancy, your heart will pump about 40 percent more blood than it did prepregnancy.
- Hormonal changes can bring about an excess of saliva, especially in women who experience morning sickness.
- Although you can't feel it, your uterus begins expanding, growing from the size of a clenched fist to the size of a softball by week 8.

MONTH THREE (WEEKS 9–13)

- Your breast size increases as milk ducts and glands enlarge and prepare for breastfeeding.
- By the end of the first trimester, your energy levels should begin to rebound.
- Your baby's heartbeat can be usually be heard, using Doppler ultrasound, by week 12!
- Your growing uterus fills your pelvis and now begins stretching into your abdomen. You might be able to feel your uterus just above your pubic bone by the end of the first trimester.

Plus-Size Concerns—The First Trimester

Question: *I am about sixty pounds above my ideal weight and just found out I am five weeks pregnant. The plan was to lose weight and then conceive. Since it is so early in my pregnancy, should I try to lose the extra weight now?*

Answer: It's a bad idea to start or continue weight-loss diets when you are pregnant. Your baby's growth and development depend on the nutrients (vitamins, minerals, carbohydrates, proteins, and fats) found in the foods you eat. Dieting to lose weight at any time during pregnancy can deny your baby essential nourishment. Instead, change your eating habits to include more fresh fruit and vegetables, whole-grain breads and cereals, lean cuts of meat, "good fats" such as olive oil, and calcium-rich dairy products such as yogurt. Cut down on sugary snacks/beverages and any other junk food. If you need help making healthy food choices, meet with a nutritionist (easily set up through your provider's office) to discuss optimal caloric intake and nutritious menu plans.

Experts agree that even obese women should gain weight during pregnancy. Studies prove that when obese women lose weight or gain too little during pregnancy, the result can be a low-birth-weight baby. These babies can face a number of problems once they are born. Plus-size women with a BMI between 25 and 29 (overweight) are currently recommended to gain between 15 and 25 pounds. Plus-size women whose BMI is 30 or greater (obese) are generally encouraged to gain at least 15 pounds. According to research results, women who stay within these weight gain goals have the best chance of a normal-weight, healthy baby. Remember, though, these are only recommendations. Discuss with your prenatal care provider what weight gain goal is best for your pregnancy.

Question: *I lost 30 pounds before conceiving, going from 250 to 220. I feel more energetic, look better, and after years of trying to conceive, I definitely think the weight loss jump-started my fertility. I was ecstatic to discover I'm pregnant, but disappointed to find out that for my height, my BMI still places me in the obese category. Was all my work for nothing?*
Answer: Absolutely not! Losing as little as 5 to 10 percent of your overall body weight (and you lost 12 percent) can lower blood pressure and reduce your chances for developing diabetes. Your increased energy level is a definite sign your body is healthier as you begin pregnancy. You are right to think your weight loss played a role in helping you conceive. Studies show that even modest weight loss may restore normal ovulation in plus-size women for whom this is a problem. Even though your BMI is still classified as obese, what's important is that it's lower than before. This may decrease your risk of encountering gestational diabetes, preeclampsia, and delivery by cesarean section.

Depending on the type of diet you followed, weight loss (especially rapid weight loss) can deplete the body of vitamins and minerals critical to your baby's development. Women who were on weight-loss diets before becoming pregnant *must* take a prenatal vitamin to make up for any deficiencies. Ideally, prenatal vitamins should be started by all women before conception. As explained above, dieting to lose weight during pregnancy is not a good idea. So, if you have not already, raise your daily caloric intake to meet your recommended weight-gain goals. Eat an increased amount of healthy foods, not "empty calorie" junk foods. You can resume your weight-loss diet postpartum.

Question: *Before my first prenatal appointment, I was told to call the lab and schedule a one-hour glucose test to screen for diabetes. I thought this was not done until much later in pregnancy. Why am I being tested for diabetes now?*

Answer: Your prenatal care provider wants to make sure you are not entering pregnancy with undiagnosed Type II diabetes. Plus-size women are often screened for preexisting diabetes (high blood sugar) during preconception care or early on in the first trimester because obesity and overweight are risk factors for developing this disease. Uncontrolled high blood sugar levels during early pregnancy may cause birth defects in a developing fetus. If Type II diabetes is diagnosed, your provider will show you the steps you can take to keep your baby safe.

Before the initial diabetes screening test, called the *glucose challenge test* (GCT), you simply eat your normal diet and are not required to fast. You drink a syrupy, sweet colalike beverage (often orange flavored) and then have a blood sample drawn one hour later. Blood samples containing what is considered a normal amount of blood glucose (sugar) indicate you do not have diabetes. Pregnancy hormones often interfere to falsely produce high blood glucose results. When the amount of sugar in your blood is higher than normal after the one-hour screening, you will require the more complete, three-hour *glucose tolerance test* (*GTT*) to determine whether you have Type II diabetes. If testing shows you do have diabetes, your provider will immediately teach you the steps you should know to control your blood sugar and keep your pregnancy healthy.

It should be noted that not all plus-size women require early screening for Type II diabetes. Your provider will look at your complete personal and family health history to assess if testing is needed. It is recommended, however, that all women be screened for gestational diabetes around week 28 of pregnancy.

Question: *I was only slightly overweight with my first baby and my pregnancy was absolutely problem-free. Now 10 weeks pregnant with my second child, I am about 80 pounds too heavy. I just figured out my BMI and it is 35. Will I experience complications during this pregnancy because of my size? If so, which ones?*

Answer: Having one successful pregnancy under your belt is a good sign your second pregnancy will be just fine. However, you are correct to be concerned about your extra weight. While a majority of all plus-size women have normal pregnancies and perfectly healthy babies, medical studies show obese women, those with a BMI over 30, do have higher rates of certain complications. Among these complications are: gestational diabetes, gestational hypertension, preeclampsia, cesarean section delivery, and postpartum infection (related to cesarean delivery). Babies born to obese women have a greater frequency of *macrosomia*, meaning a birth weight above 10 pounds.

Remember, there is no one-size-fits-all rule when it comes to pregnancy. Women with high BMIs may sail through pregnancy and childbirth without a single problem. Obese women entering pregnancy with chronic hypertension and/or Type II diabetes, and obese women with a strong family history of these diseases, are generally the most likely to experience problems. Look carefully at your personal and family health history for these important clues.

Because you weigh considerably more during this pregnancy, your provider will most likely pay more attention to your blood pressure and blood sugar to make sure you have not developed hypertension or diabetes in the time since your first child was born. Your recommended weight gain for this pregnancy is about 15 pounds, a lower amount than during your first pregnancy.

You can significantly enhance your pregnancy's overall health by taking a few simple steps. Look closely at what you are eating and make sure your food choices are as nutritious as possible. Cut out any junk food and sugary snacks. If your provider gives you the okay, start taking a prenatal exercise class or simply go for a thirty-minute walk every day. Every pregnancy can benefit from good nutrition and safe exercise. Most importantly, don't spend your pregnancy worrying about what could go wrong. Instead, focus your energy on preparing your family for its newest addition!

Question: *I just had my first prenatal checkup. My obstetrician referred me for an ultrasound to accurately date my pregnancy.*

Since I know when my last menstrual period began, why do I still need an ultrasound?
Answer: For conventional purposes, pregnancy is dated from the first day of the last menstrual period (LMP). Using this dating method, most pregnancies last around 40 weeks. The first day of the LMP is used because most women know when their last period began.

At your first prenatal checkup, your provider will predict an estimated due date based on the information you provide about your LMP. Your provider will then attempt to *palpate* (feel) the top part of the growing uterus. Most women have their first prenatal checkup during the second or third month of pregnancy, and at this time the *fundus,* as the top of the uterus is known, should be felt about an inch above the pubic bone. Finding this reassures your provider that fetal growth is on track and the estimated due date is accurate.

There are a few reasons to explain why your provider wants you to have an ultrasound. Plus-size women are more likely to experience irregular ovulation, especially women with obese BMIs. Did your cycles vary in length? If your cycles were 26 days one month and 35 days the next, ovulation might not have occurred exactly two weeks after the onset of menstruation. The typical window of ovulation and fertilization might have been much later in your cycle.

Maybe you do have extremely regular cycles, but the second piece of information your provider needs, locating the fundus, is not possible because you carry extra weight in your abdomen. In both these cases, ultrasound can more accurately establish your pregnancy's due date and double check early fetal development.

Ultrasounds have not shown any harmful effects in the more than twenty years this technology has been routinely used in prenatal care. Vaginal ultrasound, rather than the traditional abdominal ultrasound, is used more frequently during the first trimester. Vaginal ultrasound relies on a wandlike ultrasound transducer inserted into the vagina to create a picture of the fetus. It usually takes only a few minutes to complete a vaginal ultrasound.

An accurate estimate of your pregnancy's *gestational age,* meaning the number of weeks pregnant, is important for monitoring your baby's health. If estimated incorrectly, signs that growth and development are off track might be missed. Certain screening tests, such as the AFP (alpha-fetoprotein) test, need to be performed at rather precise points in pregnancy. Ultrasound dating helps ensure these tests are given at the proper time. And don't forget the bonus for you—a very early sneak peak of your little one!

Question: *I am 5 weeks pregnant and weigh 240 pounds. I saw a news segment on TV last night linking obese mothers with increased rates of neural tube defects in babies. The report also said that folic acid might not work in obese women to protect against birth defects. What does this mean for my baby? I am really scared and frightened that something is wrong.*

Answer: Neural tube defects (NTDs), such as spina bifida, are rare in all pregnancies, including plus-size pregnancies. While there is no doubt that the information you encountered about NTDs is frightening, knowing what the actual research says can help put your mind at ease. Brief new reports about health issues tend to be more alarming than reassuring.

During the first few weeks after conception the *neural tube* forms one of the embryo's first recognizable features. As the embryo develops, the neural tube changes into the spinal cord and brain. Problems with this transformation can result in defects ranging from mild developmental issues to life-threatening complications.

According to statistics from 2003, neural tube defects affect less than 0.2 percent of all pregnancies in the United States. This means that more than 99.8 percent of babies do not develop NTDs. Recent medical research has looked for similarities among the small group of women whose pregnancies were complicated by these neural abnormalities. From these studies, it was found that obese women were slightly more likely to be in that 0.2 percent.

Several studies have been done to see what the odds are for an obese woman's pregnancy becoming complicated by a neural tube defect. Study results vary anywhere from 1.5 to 3.5 times as likely. This means instead of expecting 0.2 percent of high-BMI women to have babies with NTDs, the percentage increases to 0.3 to 0.7 percent, depending on the research study you are reading. The risk is still less than 1 percent for obese women. 99.7 to 99.3 percent of plus-size pregnancies will be free from NTDs. The odds are overwhelmingly in your favor to have a healthy pregnancy.

Research about neural tube defects and obesity also looked at the role of folic acid, uncovering some interesting results. Folic acid supplementation is credited for lowering the overall rate of neural tube defects in the United States over the past few decades. All women of childbearing age are strongly urged to take a daily folic acid supplement of 400 micrograms (mcg) to protect their pregnancies. But upon examination, in the relatively small number of obese women whose pregnancies were affected by neural tube defects, the 400 mcg recommended daily allowance (RDA) for folic acid did not seem to work as well.

Some obese women taking the standard RDA still had pregnancies complicated by neural abnormalities. A number of experts think this may indicate obese women need more folic acid than the current RDA of 400 mcg. Women with known risk factors for neural tube defects, such as already having a child with spina bifida, are advised to take 4 mg (4,000 mcg) of folic acid daily. Should obese (and overweight) women do the same? Studies are not yet available to back up any claim for increased folic acid intake. Be sure to discuss this issue with your prenatal care provider. In the meantime, make sure you are taking a prenatal vitamin containing folic acid and look for ways to boost folate/folic acid consumption in your diet. Folate is the natural source of folic acid and is found in such foods as spinach, broccoli, oranges, bananas, milk, and dried beans. Since 1996, commonly eaten items, such as bread and cereal, have been enriched with folic acid. Include a few servings of folate/folic acid–containing foods at each meal.

Also, avoid the more common risk factors for developing neural tube defects: illegal drug use or taking medications known to be harmful to fetal development. Be cautious about chemical exposures, especially if toxic cleaning materials and other hazardous substances are used where you work.

Though neural tube defects develop during the first few weeks of pregnancy, it is not until early in the second trimester that such abnormalities can be detected (between the 14th and 22nd week of pregnancy). An AFP test is a simple blood test to measure the amount of alpha-feto protein in your blood. All babies produce this protein in their livers. AFP is excreted by your baby into the amniotic fluid and then reabsorbed into your bloodstream. The more AFP your baby makes and excretes, the higher the level of AFP will be in your blood sample. Higher than normal levels of AFP might indicate a neural tube defect.

Because what is considered a normal level of AFP differs due to a woman's age and weight, as well as the age of the fetus, AFP testing has a high false-positive rate. Only a few women of every hundred who have abnormal AFP test results actually have a baby with a neural tube defect. When results are abnormal, you will have an ultrasound to visually detect the defect. If this has not cleared up questions, you will be offered the option of amniocentesis testing. If after further testing a neural tube defect is found, counseling about possible treatment options is always provided.

Second Trimester (Weeks 14–27)

Your Baby: A Time of Transformations

OVER THE NEXT several weeks your baby begins to look and act more like, well, your baby! Rapid fetal growth and development continue throughout the fourth, fifth, and sixth months of pregnancy. Your baby's body takes on more human proportions as muscles strengthen and bone growth continues.

Fetal movement becomes more and more determined over the course of the next few months. At some point during the second trimester, you will detect your baby's first faint kicks. Ear development advances and most medical experts agree that a fetus hears some sounds by week 26. You may even notice your baby startle at sudden loud noises.

As the brain and nervous system continue to mature, your baby begins to sleep and wake. Eyelids start to open and shut. Most amazingly, a baby born at the end of pregnancy's sixth month has a chance for survival with proper intensive care.

Milestones

MONTH FOUR (WEEKS 14–17)

- Your baby's mouth begins making sucking motions, probably to prepare for breastfeeding. Don't be surprised if an ultrasound shows a thumb-sucking fetus!
- Amniotic fluid is routinely swallowed and passed as urine (your baby is now the main supplier of its amniotic fluid).
- For those who want to find out before birth, your baby's gender is usually visible through ultrasound.
- The average fetus measures about 4¾ inches long from crown to rump, and weighs approximately 3½ ounces.

MONTH FIVE (WEEKS 18–21)
- Fine hair (*lanugo*) covers your baby's entire body.
- Some hair appears on the scalp.
- Your baby's skin becomes less transparent.
- The average fetus measures about 7½ inches from crown to rump, and weighs approximately 11 ounces.

MONTH SIX (WEEKS 22–27)
- Your baby can grin and frown as facial muscles grow in strength.
- Your baby's movements become more coordinated. Since you can probably feel your baby by now, you can detect the increasingly rhythmic movements firsthand.
- Footprints and fingerprints form. Fingernails begin to develop.
- By week 24, the average fetus measures about 8¼ inches and weighs approximately 1.4 pounds.

Your Body—Comfortably Pregnant

Most women experience a renewed sense of energy as the second trimester begins. The early inconveniences of pregnancy, such as morning sickness, tend to disappear (though a few will return in later months). The chance for miscarriage decreases. If you held off telling family, friends, and/or co-workers the good news until the beginning of the fourth month, their well-wishes can increase your own happiness and excitement. Women report feeling more confident and comfortable about pregnancy once the second trimester begins.

Feeling your baby move for the first time is a second trimester highlight and one of pregnancy's most cherished moments. Called *quickening,* the first sensation of movement is reported by women to feel like fluttering, tiny bubbles, butterflies, or tapping. Trust us, you will know it when you feel it and be able to make your own comparisons. Quickening usually takes place anywhere from week 18 to 24 of pregnancy in first-time mothers, earlier if you have already had a baby.

Common Experiences

MONTH FOUR (WEEKS 14–17)
- Your nipples and *areolae* (darkened skin around the nipple) become darker.

- Though less tender than in the first trimester, your breasts continue to grow in size.
- Appetite rebounds from first trimester morning sickness and food aversions.
- Your uterus stretches to about 1½ inches below your belly button and is the size of a cantaloupe.

MONTH FIVE (WEEKS 18–21)
- In preparation for milk production after birth, your breasts might begin to leak a yellowish premilk fluid called *colostrum.*
- As your uterus stretches in size and grows heavier, your center of gravity shifts. It is common to experience mild back pain during the second trimester as you change your posture to accommodate for your newly protruding tummy.
- Heartburn is more frequent as your uterus presses against your gastrointestinal tract.
- Your uterus is now the size of a honeydew melon and stretches to your belly button.

MONTH SIX (WEEKS 22–27)
- Time to buy some moisturizer! The result of a beautifully bulging belly is often stretched-out, itchy skin.
- You may experience *Braxton-Hicks contractions* as your uterus briefly contracts and releases in preparation for the big event a few months down the road. Braxton-Hicks contractions are not painful. Contact your provider if you do feel pain or the contractions repeat in a noticeable, frequent pattern (such as contractions every 10 to 15 minutes).
- You should be able to feel your baby by now, detecting periods of intense activity, rest, and even hiccups!
- Your uterus is now 2½ inches above your belly button and your uterus is the size of a small watermelon.

Plus-Size Questions—Second Trimester

Question: *I've noticed that a few varicose veins have appeared on my calves. What causes varicose veins and can I prevent them from spreading further?*

Answer: *Varicose veins* are a common—and unwanted—pregnancy side effect. Veins return blood to the heart for recirculation. Like the rest of your blood vessels, veins perform extra work to carry a naturally increased blood volume during pregnancy (as much as four additional pints). Tiny valves lining the leg veins keep blood flowing along at just the right speed and, most important, help blood in the legs defy gravity as it travels back to the heart.

When an expanding uterus and pregnancy weight gain place too much pressure on already overworked leg veins, valves become unable to properly open and close. Blood pools around impaired valves, resulting in bulging veins visible beneath the skin's surface. Pregnancy hormones, meant to relax the blood vessels to increase blood flow to the growing fetus, may also contribute to improperly working valves and varicose veins.

If your mother developed varicose veins, you are particularly susceptible, because varicose veins are often an inherited trait. Plus-size women are at increased risk for varicosities, even more so if weight gain during pregnancy exceeds recommended amounts.

Varicose veins are often accompanied by varying degrees of achiness, swelling, and leg fatigue. Monitor your varicose veins for any red and swollen areas that are tender to the touch. This could indicate a blood clot. Also, make sure to let your prenatal care provider know you have developed varicose veins.

It may be possible to prevent—or at least minimize—the appearance of varicose veins by taking measures to relieve pressure on the legs. Some practical ways to help blood flow include:

- **Avoid excessive weight gain.** Make sure you know what the recommended weight gain is for your BMI. Talk to you provider and/or registered dietitian about how best to pace your weight gain throughout pregnancy.
- **Don't stand or sit for prolonged periods of time.** When sitting, avoid crossing your legs. If your job requires you to sit for most of the workday, elevate your legs. Flex and rotate your ankles a few times every hour.
- **Wear support hose or compression stockings during the day.** These are available at most drugstores; they relieve achiness and help improve blood flow. At night, elevate your legs with pillows.
- **Engage in moderate exercise, such as swimming, walking, or prenatal yoga.** Exercising just three times a week can significantly improve your circulation. Always

discuss any exercise program with your provider to make
sure it is safe for your pregnancy.

- **Sleep on your left side instead of flat on your back.**
This takes pressure off the *vena cava*, the major vein
returning blood from your legs to your heart. Lying flat on
your back decreases circulation.
- **Monitor the development of varicose veins.** Varicose
veins can appear not only on legs; they can also spread
to the vulva and rectum (the latter are known as *hemorrhoids*). Bulging veins in these areas are often very
uncomfortable. For women with hemorrhoids, witch
hazel pads and ice packs are helpful in relieving pain.
- **Increase the amount of vitamin C in your diet.** Vitamin C helps maintain your blood vessels' elasticity,
enabling veins to better withstand pressure. Try eating
more vitamin C–rich foods, such as bell peppers, broccoli, spinach, and oranges.

Varicose veins will most likely fade, or sometimes completely
disappear, after your baby is born. If varicose veins persist after
pregnancy, some women opt to have the veins removed in a procedure called *vein stripping*. Be forewarned, varicose veins almost
always return in subsequent pregnancies, even for women who
had varicose veins previously removed. The best way to keep your
leg veins healthy is to exercise, eat vitamin C–rich foods as part
of a balanced diet, and take steps to avoid placing undue pressure
on your legs.

Question: *I have struggled with depression and anxiety for most of
my adult life. Since becoming pregnant these emotions have inten-
sified and my response—as usual—is to overeat. It is not even the end
of the second trimester and I have already packed on 20 pounds. My
OB only recommended I gain between 15 and 25. How can I stop
these negative feelings from sabotaging my pregnancy weight gain?*
Answer: Approximately 25 percent of all women experience
depression while pregnant. For some, the emotional ups and downs
are due simply to surging pregnancy hormones. Other women, like
yourself, enter pregnancy already dealing with depression and/or
anxiety. Hormonal interference just seems to make it worse. Plus-
size women generally have higher rates of depression than do thinner women, though the causes behind this are not clear.

Because your feelings have begun to hamper your ability to have a healthy pregnancy, it is important to get help now. Talk to your OB about your depression and anxiety. Chances are your OB has helped many women with similar issues and can recommend some easy steps to feel better. Depending on the severity of your symptoms, you might need to meet with a psychotherapist to discuss treatment options, such as antidepressant medications determined safe to use during pregnancy. Your OB can also put you in touch with a counselor to talk about the reasons behind your often-overwhelming emotions.

Pregnancy support groups, usually offered by local hospitals, might be another beneficial alternative for you. Some groups focus solely on mental health during and after pregnancy; other groups focus on eating disorders during pregnancy. Your prenatal care team can help you locate a group in your community that best matches your needs.

Don't forget exercise! Something as simple as a brisk twenty-minute walk every day can do wonders to lessen the symptoms of depression and anxiety. Your OB can suggest types of physical activity that are safe during pregnancy.

Because your troubling emotions lead to overeating, another important person you should talk to is a nutritionist. Since your weight gain is ahead of where it should be, you need to make every bite count for the remainder of your pregnancy. A nutritionist can teach you about healthy, filling, and tasty food choices that won't pack on unnecessary pounds. Some foods, such as those rich in omega-3 fatty acids, have even been shown to naturally lessen depression! A nutritionist can help you better pace your weight gain by setting mini-goals for the following weeks and months until your baby is born.

Last but not least, enjoy your pregnancy! Allow the months leading up to your child's birth to be filled with joy and happiness. If you are expecting your first child, take one last "only the two of you" vacation with your partner. If you already have children, make a scrapbook of fun family memories. Rent funny movies (there are many pregnancy-themed comedies) or just have a laugh with an old friend. Sometimes it's true, laughter really is the best medicine.

Question: *I weigh 210 pounds and this is my first pregnancy. I am an apple shape, carrying most of my excess weight in the stomach area. My Level II Ultrasound is next week and I am worried the* *technician will say something like "I can't see the baby through all that fat." Can extra abdominal "padding" affect ultrasound? Will the technician be able to get an accurate picture?*

Answer: Ultrasound tests, also called *sonograms,* rely on sound wave technology to create a two-dimensional image of your baby. A routine part of prenatal care for the past few decades, ultrasound/sonography has proven itself to be a useful tool in evaluating fetal well-being. In 2001, 67 percent of all pregnancies included ultrasound testing as part of standard prenatal care.

Level II ultrasound examines and measures key bones and organs. An accurate sonogram can indicate healthy fetal growth or potential developmental problems. Level II ultrasounds are most often performed between the 18th and 22nd weeks of pregnancy because all fetal organs are visible by this time. If any abnormalities are detected, further testing will be needed.

Ultrasounds are commonly administered by a trained technician or radiologist, though it is not uncommon for a woman's prenatal care provider or a *perinatologist* (high-risk specialist) to perform the exam.

Ultrasound technology is similar to detecting ships and airplanes with radar. High-frequency sound waves sent out from a small device called a *transducer* bounce off your baby's bones and organ tissues. Each body part reflects sound waves back to the transducer in a different way, making it possible for an attached computer to decode reflected waves and produce a picture of your baby. Early on in pregnancy, the transducer is inserted into the vagina but, during the second and third trimesters, abdominal ultrasound is used to obtain the most complete fetal visualization.

BMI and body shape *may* affect the accuracy of abdominal ultrasound. Sound waves must penetrate abdominal fat (as well as skin, muscle, and your bladder) to reach your uterus. Studies show ultrasound precision—how clearly body parts appear on the monitor screen—can decrease an average of 14.5 percent in obese women with BMIs above 36.

Women most affected are those with BMIs above 49. Researchers found body shape in these high-BMI women to be an important factor influencing ultrasound results. Ultrasounds with decreased clarity were more common in apple-shaped women, because of excess weight stored in the abdominal area. Women with BMIs less than 36, regardless of body shape, had clear fetal visualization during ultrasound.

Your provider already knows all this information, as does the technician who will perform the test. If your provider had any doubts about your upcoming ultrasound, chances are these concerns would have been mentioned at a previous visit. Determine your BMI to see if it is above 36 (and remember that BMIs above 36 only mean the *potential* for ultrasound problems). Contact your provider to discuss your worries, he or she will be able to give you a more realistic idea of what to expect.

As for the testing itself, remember that ultrasound technicians are trained to perform ultrasounds on women of all shapes and sizes. With experience, though, comes increased expertise. If it makes you feel more comfortable, call ahead and request a seasoned sonographer. Most important, relax! Enjoy looking at your baby on the monitor screen. Don't forget to ask for a picture or two. And while it might take a little extra time and effort to get your ultrasound right, always expect courteous professionalism.

Question: *I finally felt my baby move a few days ago, the end of my fifth month. Compared to other pregnant women I know, I am one of the last to detect movement. My husband has yet to feel anything through my tummy and this has been a disappointment for both of us. Are the delays in feeling movement because of my weight? This is my first pregnancy and I weigh 180 pounds.*
Answer: Those first few barely noticeable taps coming from your baby are definitely a pregnancy highlight (almost making up for all the morning sickness). Quickening, the official name for the moment a mother first feels her baby move, typically occurs between the 18th and 24th weeks of pregnancy. Your uterine muscles, not your abdominal muscles, are what detect your baby's first kicks.

For this reason, when you experience quickening is most likely not influenced by your weight. What *does* matter is whether you are a first-time mother. Women who have already given birth have more relaxed uterine muscles than first-time mothers, making them more sensitive to their baby's movements. Some women expecting their second or third child report fetal activity as early as fourteen weeks. Experienced mothers also know better what type of sensations to anticipate. What you might have written off as indigestion was probably your baby!

All women experience a delay between when they first feel the baby and when others detect movement through the tummy. For plus-size women, weight *might* play a role in making this delay a little longer. This is especially true for apple-shaped women who carry more excess weight in their abdominal area. However frustrating the delay is right now to your and your partner, it is only temporary.

In the meantime, bring your partner along on your next prenatal visit to listen to the heartbeat. This is a great way for the two of you to share a special moment. Try to be patient and relax. Keep putting your partner's hand on your belly. Within a few weeks, your baby's faint movements will be strong kicks and karate chops. Not only will your partner feel movement easily, you will both see your tummy shift in shape as your baby performs a dizzying array of acrobatic feats.

On a more practical note, once you detect your baby's movements, it is important to keep track of your baby's activity patterns. Regular fetal movement is a sign that your baby is healthy. There will be periods throughout the day when your baby is quiet and other times of intense activity. This is normal.

After the 28th week, your provider might ask you to do "kick counts" once or twice a day. These simple checks only require you to lie down in a quiet place and tune-in to your baby's movements, counting the number of times your baby moves (kicks, squirms, rolls, wiggles) in an hour, or the time it takes your baby to move ten times. The pattern of movement should be roughly the same from day to day. A good time to perform kick counts is just after a meal. The sudden increase in nutrients flowing to your baby is often enough to jump-start some activity. Contact your provider immediately if you stop feeling fetal movement or kick counts show a lack of activity.

Question: *My obstetrician wants me to consult with a perinatalogist just to "make sure everything is okay." I am a bit puzzled by this because, as I enter the second trimester, my pregnancy seems fine. Is it standard for plus-size women to see perinatalogists? I weigh 275 pounds and this is my first pregnancy.*

Answer: Perinatalogists are obstetricians who specialize in treating high-risk pregnancy. Simply being overweight or obese is usually not enough to warrant treatment by a high-risk specialist. Perinatalogists care for women with preexisting medical conditions such as hypertension and Type I diabetes, strong histories of miscarriage, or multiple-birth pregnancies. Perinatalogists also diagnose and treat fetal development problems. Women with abnormal readings on the AFP test often meet with a perinatalogist for further testing. It is normal for women to see a perinatalogist for consultation or tests only, sticking with their regular provider for the standard checkup schedule.

It sounds like you need to have another conversation with your OB about what specific reasons led to this decision, especially if your health history is low risk and your second trimester AFP and level II ultrasound tests are normal. Is your OB new to the profession? If so, maybe it's a lack of experience with plus-size patients. Your obstetrician might need a second opinion to feel confident you are receiving the best care. For OBs in solo practices, referral to a perinatalogist could be the most practical choice.

Has your obstetrician had difficulty finding the heartbeat during exams? Did your level II ultrasound provide enough visualization of the fetus? Whatever the issue, it is important for you to know why this choice was made for your prenatal care.

Plus-size pregnancy, because it can mean increased risk for certain complications, does require closer supervision. For some women, this means having an earlier than normal gestational diabetes blood screen or more frequent ultrasounds. For others, it can mean meeting with a specialized medical professional like a perinatologist as part of prenatal care. Chances are this meeting will confirm what you already feel: your pregnancy is just fine!

Question: *Because of my weight and family history, I was tested during the first trimester for preexisting Type II diabetes. Fortunately, the results were normal. My doctor has me scheduled for another one-hour glucose screening test at my 28-week appointment to check for gestational diabetes. Is this test necessary? I really don't want to get stuck with a needle again.*

Answer: Although you did not have preexisting Type II diabetes when you became pregnant, you could be among the approximately 1 in 20 women who develop gestational diabetes during the latter half of pregnancy. The same two risk factors that prompted your provider to screen for preexisting Type II diabetes—your weight and your family history—also place you at greater risk for developing gestational diabetes. Finding out if you have gestational diabetes is very important for you and your baby.

Gestational diabetes is a temporary form of Type II diabetes, affecting pregnant women of all different shapes and sizes, backgrounds, and experiences. It is a leading complication among plus-size women. Testing for gestational diabetes is identical to what you underwent early on in pregnancy. The first step is a one-hour glucose challenge test.

After drinking the sweet "glucola" drink, your blood is drawn one hour later to see how much glucose (sugar) is present in the blood sample. If your blood glucose level is within normal range, you do not have gestational diabetes. Higher than normal blood glucose means you will need to take the longer three-hour glucose tolerance test. Results from this test definitively indicate whether or not you have gestational diabetes.

Detecting gestational diabetes is crucial to your pregnancy's health as you enter the third trimester. If you are diagnosed with gestational diabetes, making changes to your diet, exercising regularly, and possibly using insulin can quickly bring your blood sugar levels under control. Women who successfully manage their gestational diabetes decrease their risk for further complications.

In contrast, poorly controlled high blood sugar levels place you and your baby in jeopardy. Uncontrolled gestational diabetes can be associated with an increased risk for preeclampsia, among other problems. Excess blood sugar also crosses the placenta, providing your baby with more calories than needed. Your baby stores this extra nourishment as fat. Babies whose mothers fail to control their blood sugar levels often have extremely high birth weights. These babies, some weighing more than 10 pounds, may suffer birth injuries and other difficulties during delivery.

Talk to your provider about your individual risk factors and how quickly you will be told the results of your test. For more about managing gestational diabetes, please read chapter 7.

Third Trimester—Weeks 28–40

Your Baby: Ready, Set, Grow!

You constantly feel your baby's kicks and squirms. Besides getting a lot of exercise, what exactly is your baby up to during the third trimester? Growing, growing, and growing some more! Dramatic increases in height and weight put some of the finishing touches on fetal development. Babies gain from ¼ to ½ pound per week during the last few months of pregnancy and grow an average of four inches.

Until the last trimester, your baby's skin was almost transparent. Added weight forms a layer of fat beneath the skin. Fat is necessary for survival outside the womb because it maintains body temperature and provides a protective cushion for the body. Gaining weight also means your baby gradually loses that red and wrinkly appearance. By 37 weeks, the skin is smooth and your baby looks newborn plump.

Milestones

MONTH SEVEN (WEEKS 28–31)

- The fetus's lungs continue to mature. Regular rhythmic breathing movements begin.
- All bones have formed and continue to grow and harden (using the calcium you provide). Skull bones become firmer but do not fuse in order to allow for greater flexibility as your baby negotiates the birth canal during delivery.
- The fetus begins to store iron (again, provided by you). Iron stores can last up to six months after your baby is born. This mineral is important for the development of healthy red blood cells.
- With excellent care and no further complications, a baby born after week 29 has a good chance for survival.

MONTH EIGHT (WEEKS 32–35)

- Lanugo hair, which covered your baby's entire body during the previous trimester, begins to disappear. At birth, you might notice some remaining on your baby's upper arms and back. This is normal and will fall out after a few weeks.
- Your baby gains about ½ to 1 ounce every day!
- Sleeping patterns emerge, including REM (active) sleep. What do you think your baby is dreaming about?
- Some babies are already turned head down in preparation for birth.

MONTH NINE (WEEKS 36–40)

- Your baby is considered full term at 37 weeks. Keep an eye out for signs of labor (see chapter 9 for details).
- The fetus's fingernails reach past the fingertips. Don't be surprised if your baby is born in need of a manicure!
- The baby's brain growth continues right up until birth—and beyond. The brain is not finished with its development until your baby is a two-year-old toddler.

- Some babies will "drop" down into the birth canal a few days or weeks before birth. This is also called *lightening*. If you have previously given birth, lightening might not happen until you are actually in labor.

Your Body: It's All about the Belly!

Just when you think your body has finally adjusted to pregnancy, here comes the third trimester! Your pregnant belly, a beautiful reminder of your growing baby, is also the source of many discomforts during the final weeks and months before your baby is born. As your belly expands, the pressure from this added weight can cause backache, leg cramps, varicose veins, and increased fatigue. You might notice more of a waddle to your walk, and something as simple as getting up from a chair might become a difficult maneuver. Your watermelon-size uterus—and the baby living inside—also place pressure on internal organs resulting in common inconveniences like frequent urination and heartburn.

You will notice a change in your baby's movements during the last weeks of pregnancy as the once roomy uterine home becomes more close quarters. Your baby's acrobatic kicks and jabs will settle into more squirmy movements. At its full height, your uterus reaches to just below the rib cage. As your baby tries to find a more comfortable position, don't be surprised to feel some tiny feet digging into your ribs.

Emotionally, you will probably experience a mixture of excitement and fear as your baby's birth draws near. This is completely normal. Try your best to relax and get enough rest (try not to let your worries keep you up at night). Take a childbirth class during the last trimester to give yourself a realistic expectation of what to expect during labor and delivery, especially if this is your first baby. A better understanding of what happens during childbirth can help keep you calm. If your emotions are overwhelming and more than you can handle, be sure to discuss this with your provider.

Common Experiences

SEVENTH MONTH (WEEKS 29–32)
- Fetal movement is strong and regular.
- The top of the uterus is about 4½ inches above your belly button.
- Pressure from the expanded uterus results in the need to frequently urinate.

- Checkups increase to every other week for the next two months.

EIGHTH MONTH (WEEKS 33–36)

- Your may experience shortness of breath due to your expanded uterus.
- The top of the uterus is approximately 5½ inches above the belly button.
- Your joints loosen up in anticipation of giving birth.
- Prenatal Care: Make sure you are tested for Group B strep, a bacteria found in the vagina and rectum of approximately 25 to 30 percent of all women. Because babies born to women who test positive for Group B strep come in contact with the bacteria during birth, there is a greater chance for an infection to develop in the newborn. Women with Group B strep are offered intravenous antibiotics during labor and delivery to lower the risk for neonatal infection.

NINTH MONTH (WEEKS 37–40)

- Your weight-gain levels off or sometimes stops.
- If your baby "drops" into the birthing position before delivery, pressure is taken off certain internal organs, and you may feel relief from heartburn and shortness of breath. More pressure is placed on the bladder, resulting in increased urination.
- Your cervix begins to thin and dilate (some women do not experience this until just before labor and delivery).
- Prenatal visits shift to once a week. Late third trimester ultrasound is often performed to estimate birth weight. Ultrasound estimates are fairly accurate (a 10 to 15 percent margin of error).

Plus-Size Questions—Third Trimester

Question: *I always read plus-size women are more at risk for developing preeclampsia during pregnancy. I know preeclampsia has something to do with high blood pressure, but what are the warning signs and what exactly is preeclampsia? I am eight months pregnant and, so far, my blood pressure readings have all been normal.*
Answer: *Preeclampsia,* also called *toxemia,* affects between 5 and 8 percent of all pregnancies. Preeclampsia is diagnosed when two factors are present: high blood pressure (blood pressure readings

140/90 or higher when two readings are taken at least six hours apart) and elevated levels of protein in the urine (*proteinuria*). Usually detected during the late second or third trimesters, preeclampsia is a pregnancy-specific condition, with symptoms disappearing shortly after delivery.

Though its exact cause is unknown, preeclampsia occurs more frequently in teenagers, and in women who are malnourished, underweight, obese, expecting for the first time, or expecting multiples, as well as in women older than thirty-five. Also at greater risk are women who enter pregnancy with *chronic hypertension* (preexisting high blood pressure), preexisting diabetes, and various connective tissue and kidney diseases.

Monitoring your pregnancy for preeclampsia is a standard part of prenatal care. Blood pressure readings and urine samples are taken at every visit. Between appointments, however, certain changes you notice in your body could be important warning signs you are developing the complication. Contact your provider if you experience any of the following problems. Common symptoms of preeclampsia include:

- Swelling of the hands, face, and feet (*edema*)
- Rapid weight gain
- Headaches and/or blurred vision
- Abdominal pain (especially to the upper right, just below the ribs)
- Decreased urination
- Difficulty breathing

As blood vessels constrict, blood pressure rises. Narrow blood vessels may not carry all the oxygen and nutrients necessary for a baby to reach optimum growth. Babies born to women with preeclampsia may be smaller than average at birth. Seriously compromised blood flow might result in intrauterine growth restriction (IUGR). Babies with IUGR have an estimated weight below the 10th percentile. Some of these babies could face health problems as a result. Women with preeclampsia may experience kidney and liver function problems or, if preeclampsia intensifies, seizures.

If you are diagnosed with preeclampsia, you will be placed on bed rest at home or in the hospital to lower your blood pressure and reduce the health risks associated with this condition.

Women with preeclampsia should not lie flat on their backs (this goes for all pregnant women). In this position, your uterus presses on your blood vessels, further restricting blood flow. Instead, lie on your side (the left side is preferred). This position takes pressure off your major blood vessels, lowers blood pressure, and allows blood flow to better reach your baby.

In mild cases of preeclampsia, limited activity might be prescribed. Your provider will give you a complete list of bed rest do's and don'ts tailored to fit your individual needs. It is important to follow these instructions.

After preeclampsia is diagnosed, prenatal checkups increase in frequency to carefully monitor blood pressure and urine protein levels. This could mean weekly visits or stopping by your provider's office every day. Nonstress tests (NSTs) are frequently performed to monitor your baby's health (see chapter 7 for more about NSTs). If the situation warrants, a visiting nurse might be assigned to collect some of this information in your home.

In addition to bed rest, certain blood pressure medications are sometimes used to bring high blood pressure under control. Following a reduced-salt-intake diet is not recommended for pregnant women and has shown to have no effect on the prevention and course of preeclampsia.

The one true "cure" for preeclampsia is delivery. If you are diagnosed with preeclampsia and it is close to your due date, your provider might decide the best option for both you and your baby is to induce labor before preeclampsia is able to intensify. In these cases, most women deliver vaginally, though cesarean section rates for women with preeclampsia are higher than for the general pregnant population. Women with severe preeclampsia (blood pressure 160/100) are given magnesium sulfate intravenously during labor and delivery to prevent seizures.

When preeclampsia is detected earlier in pregnancy, especially during the second and early third trimesters, the decision to deliver is more difficult to make. Health risks for both mother and baby must be carefully weighed. Babies born much earlier than their expected due dates need treatment in a neonatal intensive care unit. As long as preeclampsia is mild and responds to bed rest, the pregnancy will be allowed to continue with careful monitoring.

So what can you do right now to keep your pregnancy healthy? Some providers might recommend taking calcium supplements to prevent preeclampsia. Calcium plays an important role in regulating blood pressure. Researchers are also looking into the antioxidants naturally found in vitamins C and E as a way to ward off preeclampsia. Preliminary results are encouraging and further study is underway. If you are high risk for preeclampsia, discuss these treatment options with your provider.

Lastly, don't underestimate the power of a healthy diet! Poor nutrition is a contributing risk factor for preeclampsia. Malnutrition doesn't always mean someone is severely underweight or starved—plus-size women who eat mainly processed foods and few fruits and vegetables might be just as deficient in key vitamins and minerals. Healthy eating habits are crucial, especially in the third trimester. Ask your provider to refer you to a nutritionist if you need help making nutritious food choices.

Question: *My husband tells me that for the past few weeks I've been heavily snoring throughout the night. Sometimes my snoring even wakes me up! What is going on?*
Answer: You are in good company, as approximately 20 to 30 percent of all women report snoring more—or snoring for the first time—during pregnancy. Pregnancy-related snoring results from several factors. Rising estrogen levels can cause nasal membranes to swell and mucus production to increase. Difficulty breathing through the nose as well as a postnasal drip obstructing the air passageway in your throat often leads to snoring. Plus-size women are more prone to snore because extra weight, especially in the neck area, can affect breathing patterns during sleep. Snoring is usually harmless and will go away completely or lessen in intensity once your baby is born.

You can take steps to reduce or even prevent snoring during pregnancy. The most effective methods are:

- **Sleep on your side.** In addition to improving blood flow to your baby, the air passageway in your throat is better able to stay clear and fully open when you sleep in this position.
- **Avoid drinking whole milk before bedtime.** The thickness of whole milk can prevent mucus in the throat from properly draining. Mucus in the throat narrows the breathing passageway, causing snoring in many women. If you drink warm milk to help you fall asleep, make sure it is a lower-fat variety.
- **Elevate your bed.** Raising the head of your bed about

four inches off the ground helps reduce snoring because nasal mucus can more easily drain (have someone slip a few books under each leg).

■ **Keep weight gain within recommended amounts for your BMI.** Yes, yet another reason why controlled weight gain during pregnancy is so important. Eating right and exercising can help you breathe more freely while you sleep.

Countless over-the-counter products are marketed to help people stop snoring. It is unwise, and possibly unsafe, to take any of these snoring remedies during pregnancy. Always check with your provider first before using any type of sleep or breathing aid.

While most often just an annoyance for the person sleeping next to you, snoring can be a warning sign for underlying health problems. Since your snoring is severe enough to wake you up, you may have developed *sleep apnea*. Women with sleep apnea briefly stop breathing—usually for only a second or two—several times during the night. Very heavy snoring is a leading symptom of sleep apnea. Ask your partner if you ever gasp or snort in your sleep, two other common clues your breathing is obstructed.

In recent medical studies, snoring during pregnancy has also been identified as a possible warning sign for gestational hypertension. Because snoring *is* related to more serious health complications, it is important to tell your provider about your sleep habits. Your provider can refer you to an ears-nose-throat doctor, or other specialist, if necessary.

Question: *After high blood pressure readings two visits in a row, my provider prescribed limited activity with at least three hours of bed rest each day until my baby is born. My due date is in three weeks. Since I do not have preeclampsia, why am I on limited activity/bed rest? How can I prevent myself from going crazy over the next few weeks?*

Answer: Women who develop high blood pressure during pregnancy (readings consistently above 140/90), are often prescribed bed rest and/or limited activity as a way to stabilize blood pressure. Known as *gestational hypertension*, this temporary form of high blood pressure is more common in older women, multiple-birth pregnancies, and plus-size women.

The steps you take now to control blood pressure reduce the

chance for further complication. Gestational hypertension can progress to preeclampsia. Your provider closely monitors how your body responds to bed rest, checking your blood pressure and testing your urine for excess protein (a sign of preeclampsia) several times a week, or with whatever frequency best fits your needs.

High blood pressure during pregnancy, even if never accompanied by other symptoms of preeclampsia, can place your baby at risk for receiving reduced amounts of oxygen and other nutrients due to constricted blood flow. Bed rest enhances blood flow to your baby by taking pressure off major blood vessels. Limited activity—refraining from heavy lifting and straining movements—also helps reduce blood pressure.

Even with only a few weeks to go until your due date, following your provider's recommendation for bed rest/limited activity is very important for your baby's good health. If you have not already done so, ask your provider detailed questions about what activity is off limits over the next few weeks. Are normal household chores still okay? What about driving? Going for a walk? Climbing stairs? Prenatal yoga class? Is all exercise off limits? What about your job? Depending on what you do for a living, it may be possible to continue working through e-mail and phone contact. Discuss your workplace with your provider and then, if limited job duties are a possibility, talk to your boss and your company's human resources manager. It might be necessary, and prudent, to start your maternity leave earlier than originally scheduled.

Many women on bed rest fight feelings ranging from simple boredom to depression and anger. Such thoughts as "why me?" and "why can't my pregnancy be just like every other woman's?" are common. With over 700,000 women each year prescribed bed rest for at least part of their pregnancy, you are not alone in wondering how you can cope with such a limited lifestyle, even if it is for just a few weeks until your due date. There are many ways you can structure your day to make bed rest feel less like in-house arrest. Some suggestions for making the most of bed rest include:

- **Establish a daily routine.** Even if you are no longer rushing out the door on your way to work, give yourself a wakeup time. Change from your pajamas into a daytime outfit of comfortable clothes. Brush your hair. Make the bed, if this is an approved activity, and open the curtains to let in the sunshine.

When it comes time for your three hours of rest each day, lie down in a spare bedroom or have your partner set up an extra bed in the living room. Not feeling trapped in your bedroom can go a long way in boosting your mood.

- **Distract yourself.** While it is okay to nap, being in bed does not necessarily mean being asleep. Fight boredom by giving yourself plenty to accomplish each day. Finally organize all those old pictures into photo albums. Knit, crochet, quilt, or embroider, if you know how. Teach yourself if you don't. Pay the bills. Read a novel. Start a pregnancy scrapbook. Rent movies, and invite friends and family over to watch them with you. Bed rest is not solitary confinement!

- **Get help with child care.** If you have small children, you will need someone during the day to help out. Enlist your partner, or ask family and friends to come over to watch the kids. Investigate other options, such as a day care center or a nanny, if this is financially feasible for you.

- **Stay flexible.** Reduced activity and staying in bed for several hours each day helps lower blood pressure, but may also take a toll on your body. Bed rest can cause muscle weakness and increased risk for blood clots. After obtaining your provider's approval, try adding head, shoulder, ankle, and wrist rolls several times a day. Point and flex your feet. Try other simple arm and leg stretches. These small movements improve your circulation and help maintain muscle tone.

- **Find support.** If you have a laptop, surf the Net while you are in bed. There are many online bed-rest support groups. Some have chat rooms and/or discussion boards where you connect with other women in your same situation. See Resources for some of these Web sites.

Although the days leading up to your baby's birth are not quite what you envisioned, focus on what is most important: giving your baby the ability to enter this world strong and healthy. Monitor yourself for signs of preeclampsia (see previous question for its symptoms) and contact your provider at once if you detect any. After your baby is born, take small steps to gradually increase your physical stamina. Your blood pressure will be checked at your six-week postpartum visit to make sure readings have returned to normal (in almost all cases, gestational hypertension disappears after delivery). The best way to avoid hypertension in the future is to begin a healthy postpartum eating and exercise plan. See chapter 10, "Beautiful Beginnings," for more details.

Question: *I am extremely tired all the time. My mother told me it's because I was so out of shape before getting pregnant. Is carrying around all my extra weight plus my baby the cause for this complete exhaustion? Some days I can't get out of bed. I am 8 months pregnant.*

Answer: Feeling tired toward the end of the third trimester is normal. An expanded uterus and growing baby can make even a woman who once trained for marathons decide to take an afternoon nap. Fatigue is also common in women who juggle the physical stress and strain of pregnancy with such responsibilities as caring for children, working outside the home, or going to school. Needing extra sleep is a natural signal from your body telling you to slow down and rest before your baby is born.

No matter what shape you were in prepregnancy, *extreme* fatigue is cause for concern. Constant exhaustion, like not being able to get out of bed all day, could indicate an underlying health problem. When was your blood last tested for anemia? According to current statistics, nearly 8 million women of childbearing age have *iron-deficiency anemia*. Iron helps your body produce red blood cells. Lower than normal levels of iron in your blood make it more difficult for your body to manufacture red blood cells. Red blood cells carry oxygen to all your body's other cells and help you feel energetic. Reduced red blood cell production can leave you worn out and exhausted.

Your need for iron dramatically increases when you are pregnant. Almost as soon as your baby was conceived, your iron stores (natural reserves of iron) have worked double duty, providing both you and your baby with enough iron for proper red blood cell production. To keep your iron reserves from becoming depleted, daily replenishment of this mineral is essential.

During the first two trimesters, you were probably able to replace your iron stores just from iron-rich foods in your diet and your prenatal vitamin (almost all contain iron). As your baby's birth draws near, your baby prepares for life outside the womb by creating iron stores of his or her own. Your body makes your baby the number one priority, diverting all incoming iron first to your baby and then to you. If not enough iron is left over after your baby's needs are met, *you* (not your baby) will develop iron-deficiency anemia.

Don't ever let a significant clue about your health go unaddressed because you think (or your mother thinks) it's simply a consequence of your weight. Call your provider to report your symptoms. Testing for anemia involves nothing more than a simple blood test. Iron levels in the blood are usually checked early in pregnancy and again toward the end (usually at the same time as late second/early third trimester testing for gestational diabetes). If previous results showed your iron levels were on the low end of normal, overtiredness might indicate a newly developed iron deficiency.

Pregnant women with iron-deficiency anemia take daily iron supplements in addition to their normal prenatal vitamins. If your provider determines you have anemia, you will be told how much extra iron you should take to bring your reserves back up to normal levels. Your energy level should improve as your iron stores are replenished. Drink plenty of water and increase the amount of fiber in your diet when you take iron supplements because a frequently encountered side effect is constipation.

You will also be encouraged to eat more iron-rich foods, such as dark green leafy vegetables, beans, and iron-fortified breakfast cereals. Vitamin C helps your body absorb more iron, especially from often difficult-to-digest supplements. Drink a glass of orange juice to wash down your iron supplement. Sprinkle orange slices over your spinach salad for extra iron absorption. Avoid taking your iron supplement with a glass of milk because calcium actually decreases your body'ability to absorb iron. For more tips about adding more iron to your diet, please see chapter 5, "Prenatal Nutrition."

While overtiredness is commonly associated with iron-deficiency anemia, your extreme fatigue could signal other problems. Fatigue is an often-overlooked symptom of both preeclampsia and gestational diabetes. Your provider might want to check your blood pressure and/or blood sugar to see if either of these complications is the underlying cause for your exhaustion.

Question: *Now that my baby is almost here, I worry constantly about passing all my bad eating habits and weight problem on to my child, especially since I am having a girl. Instead of happily awaiting the birth of my first baby, I am full of dread. How can I make sure my daughter gets off to a healthy start in life?*
Answer: While the weeks leading up to your baby's birth are often

filled with excitement and hopeful anticipation, it is perfectly normal to experience some degree of stress and anxiety. The issue you worry about most—providing a healthy lifestyle for your daughter—is a very common third trimester concern. Every woman wonders if she will do a good job raising her child.

Giving your baby the healthiest start in life can begin the day she is born. Choose to breastfeed. Your breast milk contains the precise balance of nutrients and calories your daughter needs to thrive. Breastfed babies are less likely to become obese later on as children and adults. Breastfeeding helps protect your daughter against certain diseases like diabetes. You benefit as well, reducing your risk for breast and ovarian cancers.

Because the positives associated with breastfeeding are so numerous for both child and mother, the American Association of Pediatricians currently recommends all babies be exclusively breastfed for the first six months of life. Enroll in a breastfeeding class offered through your local hospital or La Leche League (a worldwide organization dedicated to breastfeeding support). Skilled instructors can offer many practical strategies to make your breastfeeding experience a success.

Work together with your partner to make healthy living a number one priority in your new family. Call up the local YMCA and find out about what programs are offered for very young children and their parents. Read up on childhood nutrition. Check out the local parks, taking note of which ones would be great for outings with a baby. When a family regularly eats dinner together, research shows children are less likely to become obese. Though it will be a while before your daughter is actually sitting at the table, you and your partner can start this nightly habit now.

Worrisome and fearful thoughts, however, are often overwhelming. If taking concrete steps to address your very real concerns does not lessen your anxiety about the future, you need additional help. Share your feelings with your provider. Your provider can help you locate "new mother" groups or other weight-related self-help groups that can help you work through your frustrations. Your provider might refer you to a nutritionist to discuss the specifics about what children should be eating and tips for making healthy eating a part of your family's lifestyle.

For more about the benefits of breastfeeding, healthy family lifestyle, and support as a new mother, please read chapter 10, "Beautiful Beginnings."

Question: *I worry constantly that my baby is going to be too big for me to deliver and I will end up needing an emergency c-section. Will I have a large baby because of my size? How can I tell if my baby is getting too big?*

Answer: Medical research shows a connection between babies born with high birth weights and women with obese BMIs (and to a lesser degree, women with overweight BMIs). Depending on what study you are reading, approximately 9 to 11 percent of all obese women deliver babies with high birth weights (over 9 pounds), compared with about 3 to 5 percent of the general pregnant population.

Your prepregnancy weight can influence your baby's birth weight, but is just one of many genetic and environmental factors that play a role in determining your baby's size at birth. How likely you are to have a high-birth-weight baby is affected by any of the following:

- **How much weight you gain during pregnancy:** Women who gain more than the amount recommended for their BMI tend to have babies with higher birth weights. Overweight women (BMI 25–29) are advised to gain between 15 and 25 pounds. Current guidelines suggest obese women gain at least 15 pounds. (Gaining less than the recommended amount places you at greater for risk for giving birth to a low-birth-weight baby.)

- **Your health history:** Babies born to older women (over thirty-five) tend to have higher weights. Previously giving birth to a large baby increases the odds for this baby to born with a high birth weight. Also, if your own birth weight was high, there is a greater chance your baby's will be, too. Ask your mother or check your birth records if you don't already know this information.

- **Developing gestational diabetes:** If you are diagnosed with gestational diabetes but do not take steps to control your blood glucose levels, excess glucose eventually makes its way to your baby. Your baby stores the surplus sugar as fat, leading to a high birth weight. In extreme cases, babies born to women with uncontrolled gestational diabetes can weigh over 10 pounds. Women who control their gestational diabetes improve their ability to have babies with perfectly normal birth weights.

Researchers do not agree about the exact reasons behind why obese women have larger babies. Some experts maintain that because an increased number of obese women develop gestational diabetes, it makes sense that obese women—when looked at as a group—give birth to larger babies. Other researchers, however, studied obese women who never developed gestational diabetes and still found a greater percentage of babies born with high birth weights. Their research points to genetics as the underlying cause. Many plus-size women who give birth to large babies had higher birth weights themselves, so these researchers think that maybe the link is purely hereditary. More studies looking into the relationship between maternal obesity and high-birth-weight babies are underway.

Monitoring your baby's growth throughout pregnancy is an important step in predicting birth weight. At each prenatal visit, your provider will attempt to estimate your baby's size. As described in chapter 3, fundal height measurement, the length between your pubic bone and the top of your uterus, provides some information about your baby's growth. Fundal height measurement doesn't always work in plus-size pregnancy, depending on where extra weight is deposited (if you are apple shaped, this measurement is less accurate). Your provider already knows this and will order extra ultrasounds as needed. No matter what method your provider uses, it is important to realize that this is only an estimate of your baby's weight.

Taking excellent care of yourself during pregnancy is the best way to help your baby achieve a healthy birth weight. If you are diagnosed with gestational diabetes, follow your provider's meal plan and exercise recommendations. Even if you are not diagnosed with gestational diabetes, cut out foods containing excess sugar. Junk food—candy, cake, cookies, chips, and soda—contain little nutritional value, and eating too many empty calories puts your weight-gain goals in jeopardy. These unnecessary foods can easily be replaced with healthy alternatives. Moderate exercise, once approved by your provider, is a great way to keep your weight gain in check.

If an ultrasound shows a potentially large baby and your pregnancy is otherwise healthy, you will most likely be allowed to go into labor on your own. In one study of vaginal delivery of high-birth-weight babies, 99.5 percent of all babies were born without further complication. However, other studies show women who give birth to larger babies have higher rates of cesarean section. Very rarely are large babies unable to fit through the birth canal (a situation known as *dystocia*). Your provider will carefully watch how your labor progresses and decisions about the best method of delivery will be made from there.

Because these concerns are causing you such worry, make sure to bring this issue up at your next prenatal visit. Your provider is better able to provide information specifically tailored to your pregnancy. If you have not done so already, take a childbirth class to help you feel more comfortable about all your options during labor and delivery. Spend time visualizing a successful birthing experience. Most of all, relax and enjoy the weeks leading up to your child's birth.

5

PRENATAL NUTRITION

Recipe for Healthy Prenatal Nutrition

Some pregnant women crochet beautiful baby blankets in their spare time, other women pore over nursery furniture catalogs and paint chips. When I was expecting my first child, I, too, wanted to undertake some kind of project to let me know I was already doing everything in my power to give my baby a great life. Having a nicely decorated nursery awaiting him when we returned from the hospital just wasn't enough. That's when I "discovered" good nutrition.

I read a very brief article in a pregnancy magazine about how women who eat foods like salmon and walnuts throughout pregnancy supply their babies with omega-3 fatty acids, "good fats" that boost baby's brain and eye development. I was hooked. From there, I read up extensively on nutrition and figured out the most important nutrients to eat during pregnancy and how to structure my daily meals. I collected countless recipes. Most were easy to prepare and very satisfying. I fell in love all over again with the smell, texture, and taste of food.

Eating right, really for the first time in my adult life, enabled me to feel more confident about my plus-size pregnancy and more actively involved in "growing" my baby. I truly nourished both of us and it worked! My baby boy was born healthy! The payoff for making a few basic changes to my eating habits has been priceless.

—LOUISA, age 25

- **Vitamin C–rich fruits and vegetables:** bell peppers, broccoli, Brussels sprouts, cabbage, cantaloupe, cauliflower, citrus fruits, guavas, kiwis, mangoes, papaya, orange juice, snow peas, strawberries, tomatoes, tomato juice

  One of the *antioxidant* vitamins, vitamin C helps protect your body's cells from damage. Some studies reveal consumption of vitamin C during pregnancy may prevent preeclampsia, a condition thought to have its origins in damage to the cells lining the body's blood vessels (*endothelial cells*). Vitamin C is believed to strengthen the body's immune system, helping you to more efficiently fight off infection and disease.

  Vitamin C also assists in the production of *collagen*, the "glue" that holds your cells (and your baby's cells) together. Collagen is found everywhere—teeth, skin, tendons, and blood vessels. Finally, vitamin C enables your body to more easily absorb iron. For this reason, women are often advised to wash down an iron supplement with some orange juice. Eat at least a few servings of vitamin C–rich foods every day as part of your total servings for fruits and vegetables.

- **Beta-carotene–rich fruits and vegetables:** apricots, cantaloupe, carrots, collards, greens (dandelion, mustard, beet, etc.), kale, peaches, pumpkin, romaine lettuce, winter and yellow squash, spinach, sweet potatoes, yams

  Beta-carotene is a precursor to vitamin A. Your body converts the beta-carotene from your foods into vitamin A on an as-needed basis. Eating several servings a day of fruits and vegetables rich in beta-carotene promotes healthy skin and bone growth, a strong immune system, and good eyesight in both you and your baby.

- **Folate-rich fruits and vegetables:** asparagus, bananas, broccoli, Brussels sprouts, cantaloupe, collards, greens (dandelion, mustard, beet, etc.), kale, oranges, romaine lettuce, spinach

  Folate is the natural form of folic acid found in fruits and vegetables. Numerous health benefits for you and your baby result from adequate daily folate/folic acid intake. As detailed in the previous chapter, folic acid helps protect your baby from developing neural tube defects during the very early stages of pregnancy. Additionally, folate/folic acid encourages fetal organ and tissue growth, assists your baby in reaching a healthy birth weight, and can lower your risk for developing certain types of anemia.

Because folate/folic acid is such an important vitamin, and because most women do not consume enough of it through diet alone, the American College of Obstetricians and Gynecologists recommends that all women of childbearing age take a daily supplement containing at least 400 mcg of folic acid. As noted in chapter 4, plus-size women should discuss their folic acid requirements with their prenatal care provider.

Faithfully take your supplement, but go ahead and pack your meals full of folate-rich foods.

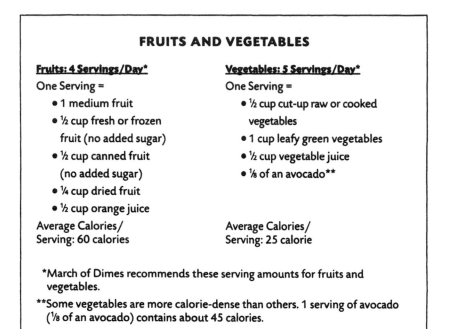

FRUITS AND VEGETABLES

Fruits: 4 Servings/Day*

One Serving =
- 1 medium fruit
- ½ cup fresh or frozen fruit (no added sugar)
- ½ cup canned fruit (no added sugar)
- ¼ cup dried fruit
- ½ cup orange juice

Average Calories/ Serving: 60 calories

Vegetables: 5 Servings/Day*

One Serving =
- ½ cup cut-up raw or cooked vegetables
- 1 cup leafy green vegetables
- ½ cup vegetable juice
- ⅛ of an avocado**

Average Calories/ Serving: 25 calorie

*March of Dimes recommends these serving amounts for fruits and vegetables.

**Some vegetables are more calorie-dense than others. 1 serving of avocado (⅛ of an avocado) contains about 45 calories.

Milk and Other Sources of Calcium

MILK PLAYS SUCH a starring role in good prenatal nutrition because it is a readily available and rich source for calcium. We all know calcium as the mineral important for building strong bones and teeth. During pregnancy calcium in your diet does double duty—it maintains your own bone density while helping your baby grow a completely new skeleton. Calcium also assists in regulating your blood pressure. Because of this, calcium (taken in supplement form) is sometimes used to prevent preeclampsia and gestational hypertension.

Pregnant women should consume at least 1,000 mg of calcium per day (pregnant teenagers need at least 1,300 mg). Each cup of milk, regardless of how much fat it contains, supplies about 300 mg of calcium. Drinking low-fat or skim milk is a good way to cut some saturated fat from your diet and save a few calories. If you are lactose intolerant, discuss adequate calcium intake with your provider. Most grocery stores sell low-lactose or lactose-free milk. Some women who are lactose intolerant are able to eat regular yogurt because it contains more of the enzymes needed by the body to break down milk sugars.

MILK

4 Servings/Day

One Serving =

- One cup (8 ounces) of milk: whole (150 calories), 2% (120 calories), 1% (100 calories), or skim (85 calories)
- ¼ cup dry nonfat milk (109 calories)
- One cup yogurt: whole (150 calories), low-fat (154 calories), or fat-free plain (137 calories)
- 1.5 ounces cheese*: full-fat (170 calories), low-fat (75 calories)

NOTE: Such cheeses as brie, feta, Gorgonzola, and Mexican soft cheeses (*queso blanco, queso fresco, queso de hoja, queso de crema,* and *asadero*) run the risk for contamination by *listeria*, a potentially harmful bacteria for you and your baby. Avoid eating these cheeses during pregnancy.

* These values are for cheddar cheese.

Unfortunately, most women fall far short of meeting the 1,000 mg recommended dietary allowance (RDA) for calcium. According to the March of Dimes, only 6 percent of childbearing-age women actually consume the 1,000 mg RDA! If your body does not get enough of this important mineral, your bones release their own calcium to provide for your baby's growth. When this happens, you are at greater risk of developing osteoporosis later in life.

Many plant- and fish-based foods also contain significant amounts of calcium, such as: toasted sesame seeds (contains an amazing 281 mg per ounce!), almonds (80 mg per ounce), calcium-fortified tofu (434 mg per ½ cup), calcium-fortified soy milk (370 mg per cup), calcium-fortified orange juice (350 mg per cup), broccoli (60 mg per ½ cup, cooked), dark leafy greens such as kale (47 mg per ½ cup, cooked) and collards (15 mg per ½ cup cooked), sweet potatoes (44 mg per ½ cup, mashed), white beans (113 mg per ½ cup), canned sardines (525 mg per 4 ounces), and canned red salmon (259 mg per 3½ ounces—if eaten with the soft bones). Because you may not eat some of these foods very often, and because you would have to eat a lot of broccoli and almonds to get anywhere near the 1,000 mg RDA, your best bet is to make drinking 4 cups of milk a priority in your daily diet.

If you do not like milk, or cannot drink it, calcium supplements can give you the calcium you and your baby need. Calcium supplements come in many different forms. Tums and Rolaids are excellent sources of calcium and can help sooth heartburn. Calcium carbonate taken with food and calcium citrate, taken at any time, are other possible choices.

Whole Grains

Carbohydrates, the body's primary fuel source, are, in part, supplied by the grain-based foods in your diet. Go to any grocery store and the words "whole grains" seem to leap from the shelves. You have probably noticed that the labels on many brands of bread, pasta, brown rice, and almost every cereal, proudly proclaim that the product is made from whole grains. Why all the fuss? Thanks to developments in nutrition research, we now know the healthiest choices for grain-based carbohydrates are foods made from grains left intact or "whole." Choosing to eat whole grains will furnish you with a wealth of hard-to-ignore benefits. Study after study shows people who eat whole grains as part of a balanced diet have lower rates of diabetes and are at reduced risk for developing heart disease.

WHOLE GRAINS

6 Ounce Equivalent Servings/Day
One serving = 80 to 100 calories
Serving Equivalents:
- 1 piece whole wheat or whole-grain bread
- 1 cup dry whole-grain cereal or 3 cups air-popped popcorn
- ½ cup cooked brown rice, whole wheat pasta, or steel-cut oatmeal
- whole-grain pita, bagel, or English muffin (each ounce = one serving)

Whole Grains v. Processed/Refined Carbohydrates

Grains such as rice, wheat, rye, and barley are multilayered. The "bran" and "germ" form the grain's outer layers. Bran is mainly fiber, whereas the germ is rich in vitamins, minerals (such as vitamins E and B_6, magnesium, iron, and selenium), and some heart-healthy oils. The

Protein

As WE ALL learned in high school biology class, proteins supply our bodies with amino acids, the "building blocks of life." Think of your pregnancy as the ultimate hands-on science lesson. Protein provides your baby with the raw materials necessary for manufacturing bones, blood, body tissues and organs, muscles, nerves, teeth, hair, and skin. Because protein is so critical for your baby's development, your need for the nutrient increases from 50 g to a total of 60 g per day. This translates into approximately six 1-ounce servings of protein-rich foods in your daily menu plan.

The average American diet contains much more than the 60 g RDA for protein. Even though we value them in our diets for other key nutrients, when you drink milk or eat such foods as cheese, whole-grain bread or brown rice, you are also getting some protein as well. Instead of worrying about including enough protein in your diet, focus your attention on the quality of protein you eat. Consider the following "nutrient dense" suggestions:

Lean Red Meat, Chicken, Turkey, and Fish

Each of these protein sources contains varying levels of important nutrients. *Vitamin B$_{12}$* assists in the formation of brain, red blood, and nerves cells, and is found almost exclusively in meats, dairy, cheese and eggs. *Zinc,* a mineral abundant in most meats, promotes healthy fetal growth. Iron from animal sources is called *heme-iron.* When compared with iron found in plant-based sources like spinach, heme-iron is much easier for the body to absorb. Meats also contain *magnesium,* a mineral that helps regulate blood sugar levels in the body. Keep all meats refrigerated and cook them thoroughly to kill harmful bacteria such as salmonella.

Fish deserves a special mention because several types (such as salmon) contain a relatively high content of polyunsaturated fats called *omega-3 fatty acids.* Also found in such foods as walnuts, flaxseed oil, and enriched eggs (see below), omega-3 fatty acids are known as *essential fats* because they assist your body in carrying out certain basic functions. During pregnancy and while breastfeeding, the omega-3 fatty acids in your diet are essential for both you and your baby. They assist in hormone production and play a significant role in your baby's brain and eye development. Some studies show omega-3 even reduces your risk of developing postpartum depression. In addition, they are important in the prevention of heart disease.

PROTEIN

6 Ounce Equivalent Servings/Day
One serving = 55 to 100 calories
Serving Equivalents:
- 1 egg
- 1 ounce cooked chicken or turkey (a standard serving = 3 ounces)
- 1 ounce lean red meat (a standard serving = 3 ounces)
- 2 tablespoons peanut butter
- ½ cup cooked dried beans
- ¼ cup hummus
- 1 ounce nuts or seeds (include at least 5 servings per week)
- 1 ounce cooked salmon, pollock, catfish (limit fresh fish to 12 ounces/week), shrimp, or canned light tuna or salmon (a standard serving = 3 ounces)

However, including fish in your diet during pregnancy carries with it an important health safety warning. Certain types of fish are contaminated with high levels of mercury, a toxic substance found in the environment as the result of industrial pollution. When ingested in concentrated amounts during pregnancy, mercury poses serious harm to your baby's brain and nervous system development. The Environmental Protection Agency (EPA) and the Food and Drug Administration (FDA) offer the following guidelines for safe fish consumption during pregnancy:

- Don't eat shark, swordfish, king mackerel, or tilefish. These fish contain high levels of mercury.
- Eat up to 12 ounces a week of a variety of fish and shellfish that are lower in mercury. Five of the most commonly eaten fish that are low in mercury are shrimp, canned light tuna, salmon, pollock, and catfish.
- Albacore ("white") tuna contains more mercury than does canned light tuna. You should eat a maximum of 6 ounces of albacore tuna per week.

- Check local advisories about the safety of fish caught in local lakes, rivers, and coastal areas. If no advice is available, eat up to 6 ounces per week of fish you catch from local waters, but don't consume any other fish during that week.

   Check out www.cfsan.fda.gov/~dms/admehg3.html for updates to this warning.

Eggs

Not only a good source for protein, eggs are low in saturated fats, and contain folic acid and other B vitamins, and vitamin D (which helps the body absorb and utilize calcium). You have probably noticed some egg cartons at the grocery store labeled "omega-3 enriched." These eggs are produced by chickens fed diets high in omega-3 fatty acids. For those women who don't eat much fish, enriched eggs are a great way to include this beneficial fat in your diet.

Some people worry about the cholesterol content of eggs. Eating one egg even every single day is little reason for concern. If you frequently make three-egg omelets, quiche, or other egg-based dishes, however, consider removing the yolk from some of the eggs before cooking. The yolk is what contains the cholesterol. Egg whites contain the protein.

Plant-Based Protein Sources

Plant-based protein sources—tofu, legumes (peas, lentils, and navy, black, lima, and kidney beans, to name a few), peanut butter, hummus, nuts such as almonds and walnuts, and seeds such as sunflower or sesame seeds—are good sources of protein, add fiber to your diet, and contain many of the same vitamin and mineral benefits as animal-based proteins. They do not contain vitamin B_{12}—vegetarians and vegans should take a separate B_{12} supplement. Nuts and seeds contain beneficial amounts of heart-healthy oils and should make up at least one of your protein servings every day.

Especially if you don't eat meat during pregnancy, be aware that each plant-based protein lacks one or more essential amino acid (of a possible twenty). Combining two or more plant-based proteins often produces a complete set of amino acids. For example, eating a serving of brown rice (a protein-rich grain) with a serving of beans gives you and your baby all the essential building blocks you both need for good health.

Fats

"GOOD FATS" ARE an essential part of any healthy pregnancy diet. Fats make foods taste good and add calories important for weight gain. Successfully including fat in you diet requires you to increase the number of "good fats" in your food and decrease or completely eliminate "bad fats."

Good fats are not hard to find. Plant oils, such as olive and safflower oils, along with the fats naturally found in avocados, nuts, and seeds, provide your body with heart-healthy monounsaturated and/or polyunsaturated fats. Good fats boost your levels of *HDL (high-density lipoprotein)* cholesterol and decreases the amount of *LDL (low-density lipoprotein)*. A higher ratio of HDL can place you at lower risk for heart attack and stroke.

Good fats are also "good for your pregnancy" fats. Plant oils are rich sources of vitamin E, another one of the powerful antioxidant vitamins. Along with vitamin C, vitamin E intake is thought to play a key role in preventing preeclampsia. And, as previously described, omega-3 fatty acids are good fats offering many health benefits during pregnancy and after delivery.

GOOD FATS

6 Teaspoon Equivalents/Day
One serving = 45 calories
Serving Sizes
- ⅛ avocado
- 1 teaspoon plant oil
- 1 teaspoon liquid oil–based margarine
- 1 teaspoon regular mayonnaise, or 1 tablespoon reduced-fat mayonnaise
- 1 tablespoon oil-based salad dressing, or 2 tablespoons "light" oil-based salad dressing

---

BAD FATS

Avoid these fats:
- trans fatty acid (hydrogenated fats/oils)
- saturated fat

BAD FAT #1: TRANS FATS

Trans fats (trans fatty acids) are liquid plant oils chemically altered to become solid, creamy fat at room temperature. The process of going from liquid oil to solid fat is called hydrogenation. Trans fats are listed on food ingredient labels as hydrogenated or partially hydrogenated oils. Food manufacturers like using trans fats because products made with solid fat have a longer shelf life than those containing liquid oils.

Trans fats are readily found in certain brands of packaged and prepared foods like stick margarine, solid vegetable shortening, doughnuts, crackers, cookies, potato chips, peanut butter (except for natural peanut butter), cakes, pies, some breads, and fast foods fried in hydrogenated fat. Why are trans fats so bad for you? Some of the many reasons why trans fats are best avoided include:

- Consuming too many trans fats during pregnancy is linked with an increased risk for preeclampsia. Trans fats can cause inflammation in blood vessel walls. Eating too much trans fat may be a strong enough trigger for the high blood pressure, swelling, and other symptoms of preeclampsia to begin.
- Trans fats can raise harmful LDL cholesterol levels and lower good HDL cholesterol levels, putting you at greater risk for heart disease. Trans fats also make it easier for blood clots to form. According to the National Nutritional Foods Association, when trans fats are absorbed into cell membranes, they cause fat to become deposited in the arteries, liver, and other organs, potentially leading to heart attack or stroke.
- Trans fats cross the placenta and have been found in umbilical cord blood. Trans fats also make their way into breast milk. Your baby needs good fats, such as omega-3 fatty acids, for healthy brain and eye development. Trans fats, on the other hand, offer no health benefits for a growing fetus or newborn.

With so much media attention focused on the harmful effects of trans fats and because food labeling now requires trans fats in food products to be clearly listed (as of 2006), many companies are changing recipes and going back to liquid oil. Some continue to use trans fats, so label reading is a must! Remember, too, where there's smoke, there's usually fire. Trans fats are most likely found in foods that contain too much sugar, salt, and refined flour. Instead of eating processed snack food—in which trans fats are common ingredients—choose a healthier alternative, such as brown rice cakes and natural peanut butter or fruit.

BAD FAT #2: SATURATED FATS

Saturated fats are found mainly in animal products, such as butter, milk, and meats. Eating too many saturated fats has been shown to raise harmful LDL cholesterol levels, increasing the risk for heart attack and stroke. Reducing saturated fat in your diet is not too difficult. Replace the butter in your diet with a liquid plant oil, such as olive oil; for baking, try oils with a lighter flavor, such as safflower oil. Choose lean cuts of meat and trim the fat from pieces of beef and pork before cooking; do not cook with lard or chicken fat. Drink lower-fat milk. Eat skinless chicken, or cook chicken with the skin on and remove it before eating.

Putting It All Together

OKAY, SO HOW do you take all these recommendations and actually make a daily menu from it? Here's how one sister turned the basic food groups into satisfying, tasty meals and snacks:

Louisa, age 25

Prepregnancy BMI: 40

Occupation: Computer Programmer

Target Calories: 2000/day

Louisa's Story: I was happily surprised by how easy it was to "tweak" what I was already eating into a more pregnancy-friendly version. The biggest change for me was switching to whole grains. I had no idea how much refined flour and white rice I was eating until I started paying such close attention to my food choices. I restocked with whole grains and quickly found out they were much tastier and filling than what I had been eating. Quinoa was a most pleasant discovery. It cooks fast—about 15 minutes—and can be served instead of rice. After a long day at work it was nice to still be able to fix a quick meal. My salmon dinner takes less than a half-hour to prepare.

- **Breakfast: Filling Oatmeal**
  - 2 Grains: 1 cup slow-cooked (not instant) plain oatmeal
  - 1 Milk: 1 cup low-fat milk (used to cook oatmeal)
  - 1 Protein: 1 ounce slivered almonds
  - 1 Fruit: 1 peach (diced—put in the oatmeal as it cooks to soften the peach and let the natural juice sweeten the oatmeal)
  - 1 Fruit: ½ cup fresh-squeezed orange juice, diluted with seltzer water to make 2 cups

continued

- **AM Snack: Smoothie**
  Blend together:
  1 Milk: 1 cup low-fat milk
  1 Fruit: ½ cup sliced strawberries
  1 Fruit: 1 small banana
  (Louisa's note: This snack actually replaced my ritual of drinking a can of soda midmorning. Even though it's been a year since I had my baby, I still have this smoothie instead of the soda!)

- **Lunch: Hummus and Veggie Pita Sandwich**
  2 Grains: ½ (2 ounces) large whole wheat pita
  1 Protein: ¼ cup hummus
  1 Vegetable: 1 cup baby spinach
  ½ Vegetable: tomato slices (about ¼ cup)
  ½ Vegetable: green bell pepper (sliced, about ¼ cup)
  1 Vegetable: ½ cup matchstick carrots
  1 Fruit: 1 Granny Smith apple
  1 Milk: 1 cup low-fat milk

- **Afternoon Snack: Vitamin C Boost**
  1 Fruit: 1 orange
  1 Fruit: 1 kiwi

- **Dinner: Salmon with Squash and Rice, Garden Salad with Dressing, Yogurt for Dessert**
  4 Proteins: 4 ounces pan-cooked salmon (seasoned with dill and pepper)
  2 Vegetables: 1 cup sliced yellow squash
  4 Fats: 4 teaspoons olive oil (used to pan-cook the salmon and stir-fry the squash)
  2 Grains: 1 cup quinoa (cooked in vegetable broth)
  1 Vegetable: 1 cup spinach
  2 Vegetables: 1 cup assorted cut vegetables (carrots, cucumbers, tomato, green bell pepper)
  2 Fats: 2 tablespoons balsamic vinaigrette
  1 Milk: ½ cup plain yogurt
  1 Fruit: ½ cup blueberries

- **PM Snack: Peanut Butter and Crackers**
  1 Protein: 2 tablespoons natural peanut butter
  1 Grain: 7 whole-grain crackers (trans fat–free)

Creating Healthy Menu Plans

NOW THAT YOU have all the basics for what kinds of foods are good to eat during pregnancy, use the following strategies to customize healthy, sensible menu plans that meet your nutritional needs and fit your lifestyle:

Eat Small Meals and Snacks

Eating frequently throughout the day (6 mini-meals or 3 meals plus 3 smaller snacks) provides a steady stream of nutrients to your baby and prevents you from feeling hungry. Eating six times a day can keep your blood sugar levels in better balance, making it less likely for you to experience fatigue from blood sugar levels falling too low. Not feeling hungry makes overeating at your next meal less of a temptation.

Spreading meals and snacks throughout the day is often surprising to family members who associate any kind of diet with going long stretches without eating. When presented with this formula for eating every few hours, many women report even the most reluctant family members are willing to give this new way of scheduling meals a try. Louisa's menu is a great example of controlled eating throughout the day.

Organize Your Menu by Week

Take some time to sit down and plan out your weekly menu. Many women like doing this on the weekend when the grocery store sales circulars arrive in the mail but, whenever you have time in your busy week, make room for this important task. Jot down menu ideas as they roll off the top of your head—vegetable omelets for breakfast on Monday, cereal on Tuesday . . . salmon and spinach for dinner one night, chicken and broccoli the next. . . . Do this until you have the entire week planned out. Then go back with an eye on nutrients.

Does your menu plan include enough daily servings of fruits and vegetables? Do you include servings from those high in vitamin C, beta-carotene, and folate? Does your menu plan include enough milk? Are you getting the right types of fat? You get the idea. Analyze your menu plan and make adjustments so that your daily servings for all nutrients are met and your overall weekly menu is healthy and balanced.

When you finish planning, type up the final weekly menu on your computer or write it in chart form on a piece of paper. Post the menu prominently on the refrigerator. This is an easy reference when you are packing your lunch or preparing a shopping list. Some women report that checking off each meal as the week progresses gives them a great feeling of satisfaction.

Family-friendly tip: Family members will eat these foods, too. Make sure your family plays a part in planning the weekly menu by giving each person a chance to create a day's worth of meals and snacks (provide some nutritional guidance as needed). Sharing responsibility for what everyone eats can go a long way in motivating family members to stick with a healthier meal plan.

Avoid "Portion Distortion"

The restaurant industry quickly figured out a great way to keep customers coming back again and again: give people a lot of food at relatively low prices. As a result, casual dining restaurants offer giant hamburgers for under $10, and fast-food chains resort to "super-sizing" foods and beverages to lure in customers.

Restaurant tactics have trickled down into our everyday eating habits. Packaged foods in the grocery story mimic what we see in restaurants. Walk down any aisle and you will notice bigger bagels, wider frozen pizzas, longer hot dogs, mile-high muffins, etc. Restaurants influence not only what's offered at the grocery store but also how you cook at home. When you become accustomed to your favorite Italian restaurant serving mounds of spaghetti with meatballs the size of baseballs, you are more likely to create similar dishes in your own kitchen.

All of this has led to confusion about what *portion size* and *serving size* really mean. *Serving size* is a standard amount used to identify how many calories and nutrients are in a certain food. For example, the standard serving size for meat is about 3 ounces. When you buy packaged foods, the serving size is located on the "nutrition facts" label. A *portion* is the amount of food you choose to eat.

If you decide to have a cinnamon raisin bagel for breakfast, that is your portion. If you read the label carefully, you will quickly see why portion and serving size may no longer mean the same thing. The standard serving size for a bagel should be about 2 ounces. This equals two slices of bread and is the equivalent of two grains servings in your daily diet. If the label reveals your bagel weighs 5 ounces, your serving size has shot up to the equivalent of 5 slices of bread. This one portion translates to almost your entire day's worth of grain servings and provides about 500 calories!

Experts identify "portion distortion" as a major reason why some people are overweight. You can avoid "portion distortion" by reading labels, measuring and weighing your food before eating, and adjusting your portion sizes if you find they are out of control. There are times—eating out, eating at a friend's house, or the measuring spoons are in the dishwasher—when you can't gauge precisely how many servings are in your portion. The National Institutes of Health offer an easy method to estimate serving sizes in foods using the following visual clues:

3 ounces of meat (beef, chicken breast, fish) = deck of playing cards

1 medium-size apple or orange = size of a tennis ball

1 slice of bread = palm of your hand

1 teaspoon of oil = size of a quarter

1 cup of milk = enough milk to fill an individual container of yogurt

1 serving of nuts (1 ounce) = 1 handful

2 ounces of whole-grain pretzels = 2 handfuls

1½ ounce of cheese = C battery *or* size of your thumb

½ cup of pasta, rice, cooked vegetables, chopped fruit = fills half a baseball

Use the visual clues to check portion size (is your hamburger the size of one deck of cards or five?) Cut back portions as needed. Switch to smaller dinner plates to make your food servings appear larger (the average size of dinner plates in the past few decades has increased to accommodate larger meal sizes!). While eating out, some women ask for a to-go box with their meals and divvy up their food before eating, leaving only the correct servings on their plate and saving the rest for later.

Drink Plenty of Water

With up to 40 percent more blood pumping through your system, you will need to take in about 10 cups of fluids each day to meet your body's increased need. Many foods, especially fruits, contain varying amounts of fluids and can partially satisfy your daily requirements. The remainder of your fluids should come from drinking water (water also works alongside fiber to help keep you regular). If you just don't like plain drinking water, add a splash of lemon or lime juice to sparkling water or add a sprig of mint to enhance flavor.

Avoid drinking soda and fruit juice (except for orange juice) during pregnancy. These liquids often contain high levels of sugar. If you drink coffee, you may want to consider temporarily giving it up or strictly limiting the beverage, because it still isn't clear what health effects caffeine has on a developing fetus. Some teas and sodas contain high levels of caffeine as well. Some experts say one to two 8-ounce servings of coffee daily probably doesn't pose any risk, but you should talk about caffeine intake with your provider. Because it can harm your baby's development, alcohol should be completely avoided throughout pregnancy.

> **If it is a concern for you,** be sure to check with your local health department about water quality in your area.

Reduce Your Sugar Intake

Adding table sugar (sucrose) or high-fructose corn syrup to foods is unnecessary for a healthy diet. Glucose, the simple sugar we use for energy, is readily available from whole grains and the natural sugars contained in dairy products (lactose) and fruits (fructose). We get enough "sugar" from simply eating these foods. If you do eat foods containing added sugar, or use sugar in recipes, do so sparingly—current recommendations call for less than 10 percent of your daily calories to come from added sugar in foods.

You know the drill for what to avoid. Cookies, cakes, and candy contain large amounts of sugar, add extra calories to your diet, and are usually made from refined ingredients such as trans fats and processed flour. Read labels for sugar content. Watch out for ingredients such as sugar, sucrose, glucose, honey, fructose (natural fruit sugar extracted and added to other foods), and high-fructose corn syrup. Instead of these sweetened snack foods, try a serving of whole-grain pretzels or crackers topped with sliced fruit.

Regular soda contains anywhere from 7 to 9 teaspoons of sugar in every 12-ounce can or bottle, providing sugar, caffeine, calories, and little else. One study showed that women who drank a can of soda every day doubled their risk for developing Type II diabetes. Though caffeine-free diet soda (artificially sweetened with NutraSweet) might technically be considered safe to drink during pregnancy, it does not provide the same health benefits as other fluids such as water and milk. See chapter 7 for more information on artificial sweeteners.

Most fruit juices are on this list of sugary foods. Why? Fruit juices, such as apple juice, contain some vitamins and minerals but, when fruits are "juiced," the fibrous pulp is often left behind. What you end up drinking doesn't have enough fiber to slow down the natural fruit sugar as it rushes into your bloodstream. Some fruit juices, such as cranberry juice, even contain added sugar on top of their natural levels of fructose! Drinking fruit juice produces a quick jolt of energy, but after the sugar is rapidly absorbed, energy levels plummet. If you just can't go without juice, an 8-ounce glass of freshly squeezed orange juice with pulp is a good bet and is rich in vitamin C. Some women dilute juice with water before drinking to cut their sugar intake.

What about Salt?

For many years, pregnant women were commonly placed on salt-restricted diets in hopes of preventing gestational hypertension and preeclampsia. When this showed to have little effect in reducing rates for these complications, experts rethought salt intake during pregnancy. The American College of Obstetricians and Gynecologists currently recommends that women salt their foods to taste and otherwise consume a moderate amount of salt (sodium chloride) in their daily diets.

Women entering pregnancy with chronic high blood pressure, however, may need to closely monitor their sodium intake. If you have pre-existing high blood pressure, you will most likely work with a nutritionist to construct a diet to fit your needs. Processed foods are usually high in salt content and are best avoided. If you do develop gestational hypertension or preeclampsia, your provider may make recommendations about your daily salt intake.

Take Your Prenatal Vitamin

Think of your prenatal vitamin and mineral supplement as your menu plan's insurance policy. First trimester nausea and/or vomiting can dramatically decrease the number of vitamins and minerals available through food intake alone. This comes at a time when your body needs certain vitamins, like folic acid, the most.

Taking a prenatal supplement makes up for any deficits. It is strongly recommended that all women take either a prenatal vitamin containing 1 mg of folic acid or a multivitamin containing 400 mcg of folic acid. If you find your prenatal vitamin increases your nausea, ask your provider if it's okay to take a separate folic acid supplement until nausea subsides.

You need to keep taking your prenatal vitamin during the second and third trimesters (and while breastfeeding) to help your body with the somewhat complex task of using vitamins and minerals. You need adequate vitamin D to efficiently absorb and utilize calcium. Iron is absorbed more easily if assisted by vitamin C. Vitamin C works better when you also meet your RDA for vitamin E. Make it easy on yourself by eating an excellent diet *and* taking your prenatal vitamin daily.

Your provider may suggest you start taking a separate iron supplement. The American College of Obstetricians and Gynecologists endorses a recommendation for all pregnant women to take a daily supplement containing at least 27 mg of iron. This is the amount typically found in a standard prenatal vitamin.

Plus-size women might need a separate, slightly larger iron supplement of 60 to 100 mg/day to best meet their daily requirements. Your blood count, which is a good indication of your body's current iron status, will be checked as needed throughout your pregnancy. Testing helps your provider give appropriate advice on iron supplementation.

Pregnancy Cravings

YOUR TASTE BUDS become very demanding during pregnancy. How do you indulge your pregnancy cravings while still maintaining your gradual weight gain and healthy eating habits? The key is staying focused on the specific taste or sensation you are seeking. If you crave candy, you want something sweet. If you want chips, then what you crave is salt or something crunchy. You can easily create healthy varieties of most pregnancy cravings:

CRAVING SWEETS? TRY:
- Fruit, especially fresh watermelon, cantaloupe, bananas, honeydew melon, grapes, oranges, or pineapple. Cut it up and have it waiting for you in the refrigerator. Keep an apple in your purse. Bake an apple and sprinkle it with cinnamon, or whip up some fruit salad for instant sweetness.
- A smoothie—see Louisa's sample menu for an easy smoothie. Because bananas are so naturally sweet, they make a good base for any smoothie.

- Seltzer with a splash of fruit juice: Mix ½ cup of orange juice with 2 cups of seltzer. Some women also add pineapple chunks to their orange juice seltzers for a more tropical taste.

CRAVING POTATO CHIPS OR SALTY FOODS? TRY:
- Whole-grain pretzels
- Rye crackers or whole wheat crackers (check labels for trans fats)
- Air-popped popcorn or brown rice cakes
- A handful of granola cereal with a tablespoon of salted sunflower seeds mixed in
- A handful of plain nuts, such as almonds

CRAVING FRIED FOODS? TRY:
- Healthier "fried" chicken: Coat boneless, skinless chicken breasts with an olive oil–based cooking spray and roll in whole-grain bread crumbs (you can make these yourself by toasting whole wheat bread). Bake for 30 minutes at 375°F.
- Baked "french fries": Slice a potato to resemble french fries. Spray with olive oil–based cooking spray and sprinkle on some pepper and a little salt. Bake at 450°F until the "fries" are crisped around the edges (about 15 minutes).

CRAVE YOUR FAVORITE RESTAURANT FOODS, SUCH AS PIZZA, SPAGHETTI WITH MEATBALLS, OR LASAGNE? TRY INSTEAD:
- Cook these items yourself. When it comes to rich and tangy dishes, restaurant prepared foods often contain excess oil (and not heart-healthy varieties), too much cheese, fatty cuts of meat, and MSG for flavor enhancement. And, as discussed earlier, the portions are usually way too big. Preparing these foods at home means you are in charge of the ingredient choice and serving amount.
- Use ground turkey to make meatballs, or add chopped onions and green bell peppers to your meatball recipe so you are able to use a smaller portion of red meat (choose an extra lean ground beef to cut down on saturated fat). Add lots of cut-up veggies to your spaghetti sauce. Make vegetable lasagne. When cooking pasta, use whole-grain noodles. Pizza is easy to make at home: Use whole wheat pizza dough (from a box mix or from premade dough available at some grocery stores). Roll the dough, drizzle

with a little olive oil and tomato sauce, top with a moderate amount of cheese, and load with veggies. Voilà! Craving satisfied.

Morning Sickness

MOST WOMEN EXPERIENCE *morning sickness* to some degree during the first trimester. It's often very difficult not to let this temporary state of pregnancy-induced nausea and vomiting sidetrack your efforts to eat right. While there is no cure for morning sickness, you can take steps to minimize its effect.

TRIED AND TRUES TIPS INCLUDE:

- **Don't let yourself go hungry.** Hunger can set off nausea. Eat small meals and snacks throughout the day. Keep a snack by your bedside and eat as soon as you wake up in the morning, It doesn't need to be much—just some crackers or toast to keep food in your tummy. Some women wake themselves up a few hours early, eat, and then go back to sleep. If you are up during the night to go to the bathroom, this is the perfect time to grab a small snack. On the flipside, don't overeat. Eating past the point of fullness can trigger nausea, too!
- **Eat what you can.** If certain smells, taste, or even the sight of a certain food makes you gag, don't force yourself to eat it. Most experts agree that simply getting enough calories may need to take priority over a properly balanced diet when morning sickness is at its worst. If all you can keep down for a few days are blueberry muffins and orange juice, don't worry. Remind yourself, this is only temporary!
- Avoid fried foods and other foods likely to cause heartburn (sausage, onions, pizza).
- Ginger root is known as a natural remedy for upset stomachs and nausea. Drink a cup of ginger tea or eat a few gingersnap cookies. Hopefully, this traditional cure will provide some relief.
- To fill the nutritional gaps morning sickness may cause, take your prenatal vitamin, if possible. Some women report taking their prenatal vitamins with their meal is less irritating than taking their vitamin on an empty stomach.

Decide what works best for you. If a certain food is appealing, try it.

Think Outside the Supermarket

Buy Local Produce

Locally grown fruits and vegetables are fresher than the same varieties shipped in from far away. Less time from "farm to table" means produce is eaten when taste and vitamin/mineral contents are at their peak. If you need to include more fruits and vegetables in your menu planning, just tasting one juicy tomato or succulent peach is enough to get motivated. Locally grown fruits and vegetables are often available at your neighborhood grocery store.

Attending farmers' markets is one of the best ways to scout out locally grown fruits and vegetables. Farmers' markets provide a tantalizing variety of the fruits and vegetables that thrive in your local area. Take your partner with you when you go and, if you already have other children, farmers' markets are the perfect place to turn kids on to fruits and vegetables. It's a relief to say, "Okay, pick whatever you want" and not worry about the results. More elaborate farmers' markets even have petting zoos with farm animals and live music to enhance your produce-buying experience. Wouldn't it be great if your family begged you to take them shopping for fruits and vegetables?

For women who receive government assistance for purchasing food, don't think you are shut out from buying local produce. Many farmers' markets accept WIC and food stamps. Contact the social services department in your area to find out which local farmers' markets participate in government food assistance programs.

Grow Your Own

If you garden at home, then you already know how much tastier fresh-picked fruits and vegetables are compared to what is usually available at the grocery store. You can safely continue to garden throughout pregnancy, with a few modifications. Always wear gloves while gardening, and afterward wash hands thoroughly to avoid contact with animal feces (especially cat feces—carrier of the harmful bacteria, *toxoplasmosis*). Do not garden in areas you know are contaminated with cat feces. Avoid using chemical pesticides and fertilizers.

Get your family involved with gardening. It's useful to have others around to physically help you garden, and your kids might be more likely to eat their vegetables if they had a hand in growing them.

Want to garden but don't have room? Herb gardens are easy to grow on windowsills and add healthy flavor to your foods. Some people living in more urban areas have great success with container gardens. This can be as simple as placing a few five gallon buckets on your back porch and filling them with soil and tomato plants.

Many towns and cities have community gardens for people who want to grow their own fruits and vegetables but lack lawn space. Expect to pay a small fee to cover watering. Call your local parks and recreation department to find out about available programs.

Meal Management

At Home

If you want to entice a reluctant spouse or unwilling children to eat the foods on your menu plan, enlist their help to cook meals and prepare snacks. Keep it fun—play music, chat about what you did that day, and give the foods you are making funny names ("gobbler deluxe" instead of turkey sandwich). Taking part in making dinner or the next day's lunches, washing and cutting up vegetables, assembling sandwiches, and baking homemade bread are fun ways to get excited about healthy eating. Besides, how can they say no to their own creations?

Share as many meals together as possible. If you are expecting your first child, this gives you some peaceful together time with your partner, establishes a positive family routine, and talking to someone during a meal slows down the rate at which you eat. It takes a while (about twenty minutes) for our brains to register we are eating. Once it does, we begin feeling satisfied and full. When you eat slowly, your brain catches up with you before the meal is through. If the "I'm full" signal kicks in before the meal is over, it's much easier to leave some food on your plate or avoid second helpings. Your contented tummy means you are more likely to stick with a light dessert, such as an apple, rather than indulging in something heavier. The old adage "put your fork down between bites" is much easier to do if you are chatting with your friends and family.

Eating Out

How can you enjoy eating out without worrying your entrée is going to wreck your weekly weight-gain goal? Following a healthy eating plan during pregnancy does not mean you are banned from eating in restaurants. Paying attention to restaurant portion sizes and food quality, however, means your good eating habits remain intact.

Preparation is key. Look up the Web site of your favorite restaurants and browse the menu online. Jot down what looks sensible to order. Check the serving sizes and nutritional information to make sure your choices contain a good balance of nutrients and calories.

No Web site? You can call ahead and ask about healthy food choices and nutritional content—or ask when you arrive at the restaurant. By law, eating establishments should have readily available nutritional information. Some progressive eating establishments make it simple and list calories and ingredients right on the menu!

When you order, avoid foods containing MSG or too much sodium, and those likely to contain partially hydrogenated oils (trans fats). Pick menu items listed as baked or broiled instead of fried. Ask that sauces and dressings be served on the side, so you can control how much goes onto your plate. Opt for a side of veggies and skip the french fries. When the food arrives, go on "portion patrol" to make sure you are not eating too much.

At Work

No matter how busy your schedule and hectic your line of work, eating right while on the job provides a constant stream of high-quality nutrients to keep you feeling energetic throughout the day. What kinds of foods should you bring? Whole-grain carbohydrates are good sources for slow-burning energy. Eat a slice of whole wheat bread with peanut butter as a midmorning snack. If your line of work makes a "sit-down" snack impossible, munch on a Granny Smith apple and a handful of almonds. Pack a sandwich, cut-up veggies and hummus, and yogurt cup for a nourishing lunch.

If you have access to a mini-fridge right in your office or share a kitchenette in the employee room, you may be able to leave some foods at work—milk, bottled water, fruit, peanut butter, veggies, cheese, yogurt—to last the entire week. If your work place does not offer much in the way of employee food storage, bring our own. Invest in a small cooler chest (one you can comfortably carry) and restock it daily.

Avoid the common lunchtime temptation of grabbing a quick bite with co-workers at the fast-food restaurant across the street. Fast-food restaurants are trickier to navigate for healthy food and sensible portions, and may best be completely avoided. As described in "Eating Out" check the restaurant's Web site or ask about the eatery's nutritional info in person to see if there are any manageable choices.

If not eating out with co-workers is just too much of a departure from your normal routine, suggest stopping by a deli for sandwiches instead of the usual fast-food burgers and fries, and make your selection carefully. Chances are your colleagues' taste buds would welcome the change.

One last tip comes from a sister who faced an hour's commute each way—and who worked up until her due date. According to Sarah, "My car became my dining room. In the morning I packed a few easy-to-grab goodies like orange sections, an apple, or a few crackers and cheese cubes. I ate my snack during my morning commute. Before I left at the end of the day, I'd make a snack for the ride home—usually half a peanut butter sandwich and a big plastic baggie full of strawberries from my stash in the break-room fridge. I swear I was more energetic than ever during my pregnancy because I never let myself go hungry."

Celebrations

If you know your baby shower is coming up, your mom's birthday is next week, or Thanksgiving looms around the corner, simply adjust your menu plan to accommodate these special occasions. To help offset any extra calories you may consume, in the days surrounding the big event eat more high-fiber/low-calorie fruits and vegetables.

View family celebrations as a chance to flex your eating know-how. Use the visual clues to cut the giant piece of turkey your uncle served you at Thanksgiving dinner because, as he said, "you're eating for two," into a more sensible deck-of-cards portion. Evaluate whether the scoop of potatoes your sister plopped on your plate looks like a half a baseball or an entire softball.

Most important, enjoy family celebrations. These are precious times, and worrying about food should not dominate your thoughts. Eat until you are full and then stop. Keep yourself busy by catching up with family members you have not seen in a while. Don't worry about what to talk about—a pregnant woman is usually the center of attention at any family gathering!

Adjust When Necessary

Even if you faithfully plan your menu, adjustments might be needed from time to time. Every month, take out one week to keep track of your actual food intake and closely monitor your weight gain. Simply write down each day what you really ended up eating and drinking and at what time. Estimate serving sizes. In addition, weigh yourself at the beginning and end of the week. Look at this information and use it to evaluate your menu plan's success.

Did you gain too much or too little weight? Cut calories without cutting beneficial nutrients. Switch to fat-free milk, eat chicken and fish instead of beef (which is higher in saturated fat), cut back further on sugary foods, and increase your physical activity levels. Sudden weight gain should be reported to your provider. If your plan leaves you too hungry and you are not gaining enough weight, you will need to increase servings/calories.

Even if the weekly menu you post on the refrigerator is perfectly balanced, your food inventory may reveal a lack of one food group, too much of another, not enough of the right foods for pregnancy, or food portions that are too big. Easy, small steps can help move your diet in the right direction. The best first step might be to meet with a nutritionist.

Working with a Nutritionist

A nutritionist is also known as a registered dietitian, a medical professional specially trained to teach people about the basics of healthy eating and how to plan nutritious meals and snacks. If your own meal plans just don't seem to be working, a nutritionist can help you tailor a diet to fit your specific needs. For women diagnosed with gestational diabetes, a nutritionist will give you concrete advice about how to control your blood sugar levels through diet.

Your provider can easily refer you to a nutritionist. Many work at local hospitals or health departments, and some are located right in the same practice as your provider. Before your appointment, keep track of everything you eat and the approximate serving size for at least one week. The nutritionist will be interested in this information, because it shows what kind of nutrients you already include in your diet, and demonstrates the types of foods you like to eat. In most cases, fine-tuning the foods you already eat (choosing whole grains instead of processed, low-fat milk instead of whole milk, etc.) and adjusting portion sizes is all that needs to be done to make your diet the best possible.

Be up front with the nutritionist about your food preferences and eating styles. Do you eat out a lot? A nutritionist can give you specific tips for how to make the healthiest choices from restaurant menus. Do you have a food allergy? Are you a vegetarian and concerned about proper nutrient intake? A nutritionist can give you help with any and all of these issues. Because good nutrition is so important during pregnancy, consider your nutritionist an important member of your prenatal care team.

Special Concerns for Plus-Size Women

Compulsive Overeating

> *I was seven months pregnant and in my car at the drive-through ordering what I always did after a bad day at work—two cheeseburgers, two large french fries, and—ironically—two small diet sodas. I ordered two of everything so it looked like I was just picking up dinner to eat at home with my husband. When I saw the same teenage boy working the drive through as the night before, I even pretended to talk to my husband on my cell phone. I talked loudly so there would be no doubt to this anonymous cashier that I had only the purest intentions for wanting this food. I inhaled the familiar aroma of grease as I drove to the far side of the parking lot, a place where I knew my car would be hidden in shadow. I parked the car and quickly went to work, gulping down the food as fast as I possibly could. No, this was not some cute pregnancy craving. As much as I hated myself afterwards for doing it, I had been gorging myself in darkened fast-food restaurant parking lots since almost the same day I got my driver's license. I was not eating out of extreme hunger. I ate this way to feel numb.*
>
> —REBECCA, age 29

For plus-size women who struggle with compulsive overeating, following a healthy pregnancy diet is much more complex than simply planning a nutritious menu and sticking to it. According to the National Institutes of Health, compulsive overeating (also called *binge eating disorder*) is arguably the most common eating disorder in the United States today. An estimated 4 million people are affected—many of them plus-size women of childbearing age. Most compulsive overeaters binge on food for some kind of emotional relief. Unlike bulimic women, compulsive overeaters do not "purge" themselves after bingeing.

Likely rooted in depression, experts are not quite sure what drives some women to regularly binge on food. Whether depression causes compulsive overeating—or is the result of bingeing—is not yet known. What is known is what women themselves report. For some, compulsive overeating is a way to "stuff down" uncomfortable emotions and memories—as Rebecca puts it, "feel numb." For other women, bingeing is a way of being in control, of getting exactly what they think they want. Momentary comfort achieved during a binge almost always leads to intense guilt, shame, and anxiety. Despite this, the urge to binge remains strong.

The National Institutes of Health lists the following as common characteristics of binge eating disorder. You are most likely a compulsive overeater if you:

- Feel your eating is out of control
- Eat large amounts of food, even when you are not really hungry
- Eat in secret because you are embarrassed by the amount of food you eat
- Eat what you know most people think of as an unusually large amount of food
- Eat much more quickly during binge episodes
- Eat until so full that you feel uncomfortable
- Feel disgusted, depressed, or guilty after overeating

If you struggle with compulsive overeating during pregnancy, getting help is critical for the health and well-being of both you and your baby. Plus-size women who compulsively overeat may gain too much weight during pregnancy. Binges typically feature processed foods high in fat and sugar—foods that pack in too many calories and not enough vitamins and minerals. Compulsive overeaters who exceed their weight-gain goals are more likely to deliver a high-birth-weight baby. This in turn leads to greater risk for delivery by cesarean section and possibly other delivery-related problems.

Some compulsive overeaters are extremely skilled at hiding the evidence of bingeing—meticulously throwing away grocery store receipts and food wrappers, keeping the kitchen spotless, eating only a tiny bit during the workday. These women are so adept at covering their tracks that loved ones and others who could offer valuable support are often unaware there is even a problem. If bingeing is your deeply guarded secret, the time has come to break the silence and get help. Because nutritious eating is at the heart of a healthy pregnancy, reaching out for the assistance and guidance you need to break free from compulsive eating is now more important than ever.

Finally "getting real" and actually talking about your compulsive overeating out loud is often the first step to ending the binge eating cycle. Confide in a family member or friend you feel especially close to and who you know will lend a supportive ear. When one sister finally told a good friend about her compulsive overeating, the friend simply listened and at the end of the conversation gave the sister a big hug. Later that same day her friend stopped by with an Internet print-out of local eating disorder support groups. On the top of the paper her friend had written, "Let's go to the first one together!" This story is a great reminder of why they're called loved ones!

While you have your choice of family members or friends to confide in, make sure to tell your prenatal care provider about your struggles with compulsive overeating. If talking about bingeing makes you feel ashamed or embarrassed, don't let it make you silent. Your provider needs to know this important piece of your health profile to best care for you and your baby. To feel more comfortable when talking to your provider about this issue, consider asking a supportive family member or friend to go to with you to your next prenatal checkup. If this isn't possible, write down the pertinent information on paper and read it aloud or give it to your provider to read.

Besides personal encouragement to break the binge eating cycle, your provider can refer you to experts specifically trained to help women in your situation. You will most likely work with a nutritionist to construct a sensible eating plan and meet with a psychologist or counselor to work through the emotional issues behind your overeat-ing. Because depression is strongly associated with binge eating, you may be diagnosed with this underlying disorder. Treating depression during pregnancy is often achieved through therapy and possibly using antidepressants shown not to harm a developing fetus.

Many plus-size sisters have used their desire for a safe and healthy pregnancy as the ultimate motivation to finally confront their com-pulsive overeating. Their success strategies include a number of ways to deal with the emotions behind their binges:

- **Join a support group.** Overeaters Anonymous (OA) is the most widespread support group network of people dealing with compulsive overeating. OA meetings take place in towns and cities worldwide. OA is a twelve-step program designed much like Alcoholics Anonymous. OA is open to everyone, including pregnant women. Each week you look at a different step in the recovery process and share stories of your own compulsive eat-ing (it is okay to just listen). Most people who join OA receive a sponsor, someone who is available to call if you have the urge to binge. Your sponsor will listen to the reasons why you are feel-ing low or just chat with you until the urge to binge has passed.

- **Keep a journal.** Write down what is bothering you. Getting emotions out on paper can alleviate the bottled-up emotional frenzy that often leads to bingeing. If you had a bad day at work, detail every last problem in your journal. After you record, blow by blow, all the hurtful things your co-worker said, write down all the good parts of your day—a leisurely breakfast, seeing the bright autumn colors during your noontime walk, feeling your baby kick, your partner giving you a big hug when you walked through the door. . . . Releasing your bad feelings and seeing all the good moments in your "horrible day" may lessen your need to emotionally overeat.

  Keeping a journal may also uncover the real reasons behind why you overeat. Some women respond, "I don't know," when asked about why they binge. Writing in a journal day after day can slowly reveal what is causing underlying emotional stress. If you write constantly about events that happened in childhood or if you see your relationship with your partner or another family member coming up in entry after entry, these are significant clues about the real issues you need to work through with a counselor or therapist.

- **Keep busy.** Some women cite boredom as a leading trigger for bingeing. If feeling that you have nothing to do leads you to overeat, find opportunities to soak up your downtime. Keep a steady stream of novels by your favorite authors in your purse or nightstand. Because your hands are busy turning the pages, reading is a better binge buster than TV. Other suggested activities include knitting, calling a friend, doing volunteer work, taking prenatal classes, going for a walk, shopping, and decorating the baby's room (leave the heavy lifting and painting to your partner).

- **Don't let yourself go hungry.** Not eating all day sets you up for an evening binge. Eating the equivalent of three meals at dinnertime is not uncommon for compulsive overeaters. Always make sure to eat throughout the day so that feeling hungry does not trigger a binge. Some women report eating a large breakfast and then eating mini-meals for the remainder of the day works to keep them from using their hunger as an excuse to start bingeing.

- **Stock your house with healthy, low-calorie foods.** Keep cut-up carrots and celery available in the fridge, and place a bowl full of apples and bananas on the kitchen table. When you feel the urge to overeat, try snacking on healthy foods.

If the reason why you overeat is deep emotional hurt you have never dealt with before, your problem with compulsive overeating may not be completely solved during pregnancy. While experts report many women with eating disorders are able to put a temporary hold on their food-related issues during pregnancy, trying to adapt a healthy lifestyle free from bingeing may be a long process. The most important step you can take now is to get the help you deserve.

Plus-Size Women and Multiple Birth Pregnancy

Plus-size women carrying twins, triplets, or quads have different nutritional needs during pregnancy. If you are pregnant with multiples, your weight-gain goals are increased. Women with overweight BMIs are recommended to gain between 35 and 45 pounds when pregnant with twins. Women with obese BMIs are recommended to gain between 30 and 40 pounds. Plus-size women pregnant with triplets or quads should discuss with their prenatal care provider the amount of weight best suited for their needs. Overweight and obese women carrying twins are advised to gain from 1 to 1.5 pounds per week after the first trimester. Steady pregnancy weight gain at higher amounts than a "singleton" pregnancy increases the chance for babies to achieve healthier birth weights.

To reach weight gain goals, you will need to increase your normal prepregnancy caloric intake by up to 600 calories a day. Pregnancy places an extra strain on the heart and cardiovascular system. While you are able to eat more calories, be sure your foods are as heart healthy as possible. Avoid saturated fat and completely eliminate trans fats from your diet. Drink skim milk, eat skinless chicken and salmon instead of red meat, and use olive oil. Use trans fat–free margarine and butter sparingly. Make sure you meet with a nutritionist early on in your pregnancy to construct a diet that satisfies your increased nutritional requirements.

6

PRENATAL EXERCISE

A Wealth of Benefits

I'll admit it. After I graduated from college I rarely took part in any kind of physical activity. My career as an accountant for a large firm left little time for the aerobics classes and power walks I had been able to fit into my schedule when I was a student. Five years after entering the workforce, I had gained about forty pounds and was completely out of shape.

At my first prenatal visit, my obstetrician recommended for me to start some kind of moderate exercise program. He explained in detail the many benefits of exercising during pregnancy. It all sounded great, but I was just too busy at work to stick with a fitness routine. Of course I didn't tell my OB this! I just smiled and said thanks as he gave me some booklets about safe pregnancy exercises. I stuffed them in my purse without any intention of actually using them.

As the first trimester progressed, I experienced such intense fatigue that during the workweek I would sit in my car at lunchtime and take a nap. Heading to my car one day, I pulled my keys out of my purse and accidentally spilled some papers on the ground. As I reached down to pick up whatever had fallen out, my eyes locked on the words "relieves pregnancy fatigue." It was the exercise information my OB had given me. I quickly read the rest. It said that if I did something as simple as briskly walk for thirty minutes every day, I might actually feel less tired. I still took my nap that day, but I wondered if exercise could really make that big a difference.

The next day was sunny and warm—a good time to put my doctor's advice to the test. Instead of heading to the employee parking lot during lunch, I decided to walk over to the park just a few blocks from the office. My plan was to walk to the park, sit on a bench and relax, and then walk back. I started off at a slow pace but I soon started swinging my arms and picking up speed. When I arrived at the park, I found I no longer wanted to sit down. I kept walking and even took the long way back to work. That wonderful sensation of physical exhilaration— something I hadn't experienced in years—soon replaced my exhaustion. My heart was pumping, my face was flushed, and I felt great.

I walked almost every day for the rest of my pregnancy and even joined a gym so I could use a treadmill during bad weather. The fatigue left and never came back. Best of all, the rest of my pregnancy was problem-free. Today I'm still walking—only now with a little company from my three-month-old daughter!

—ANNE, age 27

Yes, it's true. Something as simple as a daily thirty-minute walk may be all you need to keep yourself healthy and feeling good throughout pregnancy. According to experts, regularly taking part in physical activity has the potential to:

- Relieve backache, constipation, and fatigue
- Prevent varicose veins
- Aid in a better night's sleep
- Physically prepare your body for the hard work of childbirth
- Reduce your chances for an episiotomy, cesarean section, or forceps delivery
- Improve your mood
- Enhance your cardiovascular fitness
- Strengthen your muscles and improve your posture
- Cut your risk for gestational diabetes by as much as 50 percent
- Manage blood sugar levels if you do have gestational diabetes
- Make you one-third less likely to develop preeclampsia or gestational hypertension
- Help your body burn more calories and make it easier to reach your weight-gain goals

Because you are pregnant, you need to pay very close attention to how much and what kind of exercise you take part in, and how your body responds to physical exertion. This chapter explains prenatal exercise's most important dos and don'ts, including why you need to talk to your provider before undertaking any kind of prenatal exercise regime, how to pick safe and effective fitness activities, and basic stretches and strengthening exercises to tone your body and relieve back pain. If finding time for physical activity in your busy day seems impossible, you will find plenty of tips for incorporating physical activity into your everyday lifestyle.

Is Exercise Safe for Your Pregnancy?

Before you splurge on a new pair of sneakers, first talk to your provider about whether or not exercise is safe for your plus-size pregnancy. Certain complications may make physical exertion during pregnancy off limits. According to the American College of Obstetricians and Gynecologists, pregnant women who experience any of the following health conditions should refrain from fitness activities:

- Preeclampsia or gestational hypertension
- Prematurely dilated cervix (incompetent cervix)
- Placenta previa
- Vaginal bleeding
- Baby diagnosed with intrauterine growth restriction (IUGR)
- Preterm labor during current pregnancy (common in multiple-birth pregnancies)
- Ruptured membranes
- Heart disease
- Lung disease

Before you get the green light to begin a fitness routine, your provider will want to know how physically active you were before becoming pregnant. If you took part in a low-impact aerobics class or regularly walked, swam, biked, or jogged, you will most likely be able to continue with these activities. For plus-size women who did not exercise very much—or not at all—before becoming pregnant, and for obese women with BMIs over 40, your provider might recommend for you to start very slowly by walking or riding a stationary bike for ten to fifteen minutes a few times per week. As your body becomes more accustomed to exercise, you will be able to increase the duration and intensity of your workout.

A Prenatal Workout

A GOOD PRENATAL workout includes up to thirty minutes of a pregnancy-safe aerobic activity. Aerobic exercise raises your heart rate, increases oxygen flow in your blood, strengthens your heart muscle and lungs, and burns calories. The best pregnancy-friendly choices for your thirty minutes of aerobic activity include:

Walking

Walking during pregnancy is an easy way to become aerobically active. Create a walking route through your neighborhood, walk at the mall, or use the local high school's track. Join a gym and use the treadmill, or buy a treadmill to exercise at home. If you are a beginner to fitness walking, start slowly and gradually add minutes and intensity to your walk. To avoid trips and falls, don't walk anywhere wet or icy. Wear supportive sneakers, and make sure your laces are tied before heading out.

Lap Swimming and Water Aerobics

Water exercise provides a great workout for pregnant women. Because water helps support your weight, swimming and water aerobics classes take pressure off your back and joints. Pregnant women who suffer from back pain might find swimming provides them with some relief. Exercising in water also burns more calories than many land-based exercises. When you swim or do water aerobics, you move against the resistance of the water and expend more energy (calories) to stay in motion.

Some hospitals have their own fitness centers; your health insurance might completely or partially cover the cost of pool access at these facilities. Check your insurance policy to see if you qualify for a discount at health clubs or YMCAs in your area. If not, many health clubs offer a lower monthly rate for pool-only privileges.

Stationary Bike

If you like biking, consider switching to a stationary bike for your prenatal workouts to avoid falling. Newer stationary bikes are very high-tech and provide readouts of your heart rate, miles biked, and calories burned. You can program the amount of time you wish to bike and the kind of "trip" you want to take. The bike automatically adjusts its difficulty level to simulate hills. Those who already own a regular bicycle can purchase a relatively inexpensive stand and temporarily convert it into a stationary model.

Low-Impact Aerobics

Low-impact aerobics provides a healthy cardiovascular workout without the jarring moves and jumps of high-impact aerobics. Because one foot always remains on the floor, you are less likely to trip and fall. If you participate in an aerobics class or use an aerobics video at home, choose one specifically designed for pregnant women. Keep track of your heart rate and exertion level while you exercise.

AEROBIC EXERCISE DO'S AND DON'TS

- **Always warm up and cool down.** As you begin your aerobic exercise of choice, walk, swim, or bike slowly for five minutes to gradually increase blood flow to muscles and ready ligaments and tendons for the work they are about to do (aerobics classes have a built-in warm-up). Warming up is especially important during pregnancy because your joints and ligaments are naturally looser and as a result more susceptible to injury if not properly prepared for exercise.

  End your workout with a five-minute cooldown. Slowly decrease your pace and intensity. Cooling down helps to gradually bring your heart rate back to its preexercise state. Because you are not abruptly stopping your workout, you are less likely to experience faintness and dizziness from a sudden drop in blood pressure. End your cool down by doing a few stretching exercises to ward off muscle stiffness and soreness (see next section for stretching suggestions).

- **Stay hydrated.** Drinking water before, during, and after your workout replaces water loss from perspiration and helps prevent overheating and dehydration. Always bring a water bottle along—even if you go swimming. Because you are already wet, it is sometimes easy to miss the fact that water aerobics and swimming laps still makes you sweat. Keep a water bottle placed in a convenient poolside location and drink as needed.

- **Monitor your heart rate and exertion level.** While aerobic activity is designed to give your heart muscle a workout, exercising at too high an intensity level may divert necessary blood and oxygen flow away from your baby. Use these methods to determine whether or not you are safely within your target intensity zone:

- *Talk test:* You should be able to carry on a conversation or sing along with music while exercising. If you can't, go into cooldown mode.
- *Heart rate/pulse:* Keep your heart rate below 140 beats per minute while exercising. Take frequent pulse checks every five to ten minutes and decrease your intensity level if your heart rate is too high (take your pulse for 10 seconds and then multiply by 6). If you are used to working out, discuss with your provider a healthy target heart rate to best meet your needs. Active women may be able to safely exercise at higher heart rates.
- *Rating of perceived exertion (RPE):* Perceived exertion is how hard you think your body is working during exercise. Your rating is based on the physical sensations you experience during your workout, including increased heart and breathing rates, increased sweating, and muscle fatigue. Your exertion rating may provide a fairly good estimate of your actual heart rate during physical activity. During aerobic activity, pregnant women should aim for a perceived exertion level of 5 (somewhat hard). If you are below this range, increase the intensity of your workout. If your perceived exertion is 6 or higher, slow down and rest.

SCALE OF PERCEIVED EXERTION

1: No exertion at all (how you feel when lying down)

2: Very, very easy

3: Very easy (walking slowly)

4: Fairly easy (walking at a normal pace)

5: Somewhat hard (slightly out of breath, perspiring, but can still talk or sing)

6: Hard (more difficult to talk and you are becoming fatigued)

7: Very hard (very strenuous and you are very fatigued)

8: Very, very hard

9: Maximum exertion

- **Don't turn up the heat.** According to the American College of Obstetricians and Gynecologists, your temperature (taken under the arm) should be less than 101°F after exercising. Prolonged overheating may harm your baby. Avoid exercising if you are running a fever, and wait until after your baby is born to relax in the hot tub or sauna.
- **Make adjustments as pregnancy progresses.** If you have worked your way up to a forty-five-minute power walk, don't be surprised if midway through the third trimester your body aches from your normal routine. Listen to your body. Due to the tremendous physical strain that typically accompanies the third trimester, you may feel tired after only a few minutes of exercise. Avoid overexertion. Slow down and rest as much as you need to during the last few weeks of your pregnancy.
- **Dress for exercise success.** Wear lightweight, comfortable clothing to allow for maximum movement and to help you avoid overheating. If you exercise in cooler weather, dress in layers so you can remove clothing when you start to feel too warm. Make sure your bra fits well and provides good support for your breasts. Some companies sell maternity sports bras and plus-size bathing suits. See Resources for contact information.
- **Monitor your weight gain.** Your aerobic workout burns calories. Because you are trying to gain weight during pregnancy, you need to make sure you consume enough extra calories to maintain gradual weight gain. Current recommendations call for pregnant women to eat between 100 and 300 additional calories per day. Monitor your weight gain and adjust your caloric intake as needed.
- **Choose activities wisely.** Avoid any physical activities that could result in injury or abdominal trauma. Always use common sense and judgment when it comes to choosing fitness activities. Now is not the time to fulfill your dream of becoming the first female quarterback on the local semipro football team!
- **Consider wearing a maternity support belt.** Manufactured under a number of different brand names, maternity support belts wrap around your hips and fit comfortably under your belly. Support belts provide upward lift and mild compression to the lower abdomen. Especially if you have very weak abdominal muscles or carried excess weight in your abdomen prepregnancy (known as a "pendulous" abdomen), wearing a maternity

support belt can relieve backache during exercise and may enhance blood flow to and from your legs.

- **Don't ignore warning signs.** Stop exercising and call your provider if you experience any of the following symptoms: dizziness or faintness, increased shortness of breath, irregular or rapid heartbeat, chest pain, trouble walking, unexplained pain, fluid leaking or gushing from your vagina, vaginal bleeding, or uterine contractions that continue after rest.

Stretching and Strengthening Exercises

An equally important part of your prenatal workout is time spent stretching and strengthening your muscles. Stretching helps relieve muscle tension and may alleviate some of the many aches and pains commonly associated with pregnancy. Strengthening exercises are repetitive movements designed to tone a specific muscle group. There are countless stretching and strengthening exercises. We highlight those that are safe, relevant, and effective for a pregnant woman's body. Pick one or two to start, and see how your body responds. Keep adding new exercises as you master each movement and slowly build up to the recommended number of counts and repetitions.

EXERCISE FOR YOUR BACK'S GOOD HEALTH

Abdominal and back muscles normally work together to support your posture and body's midsection. As abdominal muscles become increasingly lax in order to accommodate your growing uterus, back muscles compensate by working much harder. Due to this greater strain on the back, more than 50 percent of all women report experiencing backache (especially lower back pain) and muscle stiffness during pregnancy. Plus-size women who carried excess weight in the stomach area prepregnancy may be more susceptible to back pain once they become pregnant.

The following exercises are simple movements to tone weakened abdominals and stretch and strengthen strained back muscles:

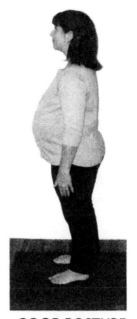

GOOD POSTURE

Your bulging belly shifts your center of gravity out from your body. Often without realizing it, your lower back is pulled forward into a sway-back posture, and back muscles become short and tight. Standing up straight is one of the easiest "exercises" to prevent swayback and avoid the lower back pain that frequently accompanies this posture.

To achieve good posture, arrange all your different body parts in perfect alignment from the top down. Roll you shoulders back and lift your rib cage. Position your head so your ears are in line with your shoulders. Contract abdominal muscles (feels like drawing your belly button closer to your spine) and flatten your back. This position brings your hips in line with your shoulders. Make sure your knees and ankles line up with your hips, shoulders, and ears. Stand with knees slightly flexed for better support and balance. Maintain this position by imagining a cord pulling you from above. Check your posture several times a day and adjust as necessary.

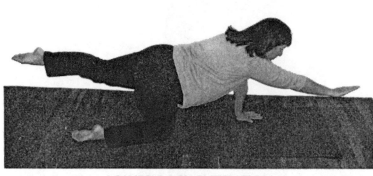

LOWER BACK EXTENSION

Extensions can safely strengthen your back muscles during pregnancy. Perform this exercise by getting down on your hands and knees. Keep elbows slightly flexed (not locked), and your back straight. Extend your right arm out in front of you at shoulder height. Extend your left leg out behind you at hip height. Contract your abdominal muscles. Hold this position for five counts. Repeat 10 to 20 times on both sides.

PELVIC TILTS

These simple movements help relieve backache, improve your posture, and tone abdominal muscles. Pelvic tilts can be done lying down on your back until the 20th week of pregnancy, down on all fours, or leaning against a wall:

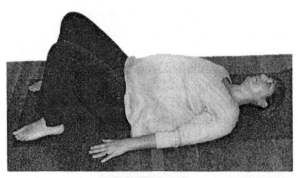

FLOOR TILTS

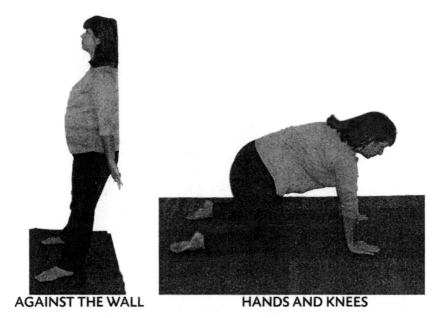

AGAINST THE WALL   **HANDS AND KNEES**

Floor Tilts

Lie down on your back with legs bent and your arms at your side. You will feel an open space between the small of your back and the floor. As you exhale, tilt your pelvis by pressing the small of your back into the floor and contracting your abdominal muscles (draw your belly button inward toward your spine). Hold for a count of five and then release. Repeat 10 to 20 times.

Against the Wall

Lean your back against a wall with your legs slightly bent. Your feet are shoulder width apart and about twelve inches away from the wall. You will feel a space between the small of your back and the wall. Press the small of your back into the wall while contracting your abdominal muscles. Hold this for five counts and then release. Repeat 10 to 20 times.

Hands and Knees

Get down on all fours. Keep your back flat (visualize your back as a coffee table) and your elbows slightly bent. Contract your abdominal muscles and rotate your pelvis so your tailbone is pointing toward the floor. Hold for a count of five and then release. Repeat 10 to 20 times.

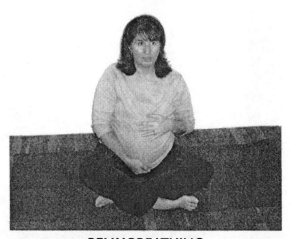

BELLY BREATHING

Sit on the floor with your legs crossed. Lift your chest and straighten your spine. Place your hands on your belly. Inhale, letting your breath expand your belly (you will feel this with your hands). As you exhale, contract your abdominal muscles by pulling your belly button toward your spine. Repeat twenty-five times. Not only is this an effective way to tone your abdominals, belly breathing teaches you focused breathing, the basis for many relaxation techniques.

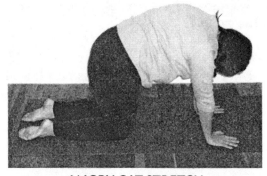

ANGRY CAT STRETCH

Get down on your hands and knees. Keep your back straight. Gently drop your head and round your back (like an angry cat). You will feel this stretch in your upper back. Hold for about ten seconds and then return to your starting position.

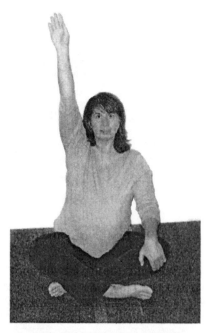

REACH FOR THE STARS

Sit on the floor with your legs crossed. Straighten your spine and shoulders. Raise your right arm above your head and reach as high as you can. Hold for 5 to 10 seconds and then slowly lower your arm. This stretch relieves tension in the back, shoulders, and neck. To perform "Double Reach for the Stars," first interlock fingers and lift both arms together with palms facing up. Hold the stretch for 5 to 10 seconds.

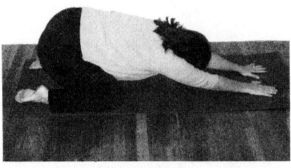

CHILD'S POSE

Borrowing a back-friendly move from yoga, kneel on the floor with knees spread apart. Sit back on your heels. Bend forward from your hips with your arms extended on the floor to support you. Tuck your chin down to your chest. Bend until your forehead, forearms, and elbows are resting on the floor. Your belly should easily fit between your legs. If not, spread your knees wider. Hold stretch for up to one minute. Breathe naturally. This is a great stretch to relieve lower back tension and promote relaxation.

PELVIC FLOOR EXERCISES

Kegels are easy-to-do strengthening exercises targeting the pelvic floor muscles, the muscular "sling" surrounding your vagina, urethra and anus. Toning the pelvic floor helps prevent pregnancy incontinence—involuntary urine loss during coughing, sneezing, or exercising—due to pressure from your uterus. Stronger pelvic floor muscles may reduce your need for an episiotomy because a toned muscular sling can more easily relax during childbirth.

Kegels

The maneuver is simple: squeeze your vaginal muscles and consciously pull them upward toward your baby. This motion feels as if you are stopping the flow of urine. Keep buttocks and abdominal muscles relaxed. Hold your pelvic floor muscles in the contracted position for three seconds and then release. Repeat 10 to 20 times at least three times a day.

SQUATTING

Squatting strengthens your thigh, hip, and butt muscles and pre-pares your body for the possibility of laboring upright during childbirth.

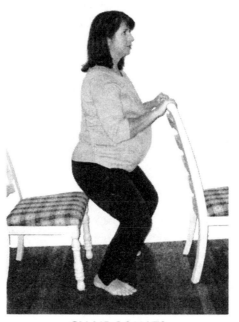

CHAIR SQUATS

You will need two kitchen chairs to perform this exercise. Move one chair so that its back is facing you. The other chair is behind you. Stand with your feet shoulder-width apart and angle your feet outward. Place your hands on the back of the chair for balance. Keeping your back straight, slowly bend your knees. Squat until your buttocks almost touch the chair. Pause for a moment and allow your quadriceps (thigh) and gluteal (buttock) muscles to fully support your weight. Slowly push upward with your legs until you resume the standing position. Repeat this motion ten times.

Note: When you first begin this exercise, you may be able to only slightly bend your knees. As you become more accustomed to squat-ting, holding the squat should become easier.

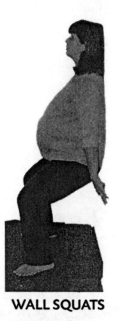

WALL SQUATS

Stand with your head, shoulders, and back against a wall. Position your feet twelve to twenty-four inches feet away from the wall, shoulder-width apart. Press your lower back into the wall and bend your knees, sliding your body down the wall as though you are going to sit down. To keep your balance, only bend your knees slightly and slide down the wall a total of two to four inches. Hold this squat for a count of five and then slowly rise, keeping your back in contact with the wall. Repeat ten times.

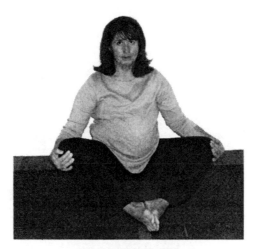

TAILOR'S PRESS

Sit on the floor and position legs so that the soles of your feet are touching. Pull your feet inward as close to your body as feels comfortable. Hook your right hand under your right knee and your left hand under your left knee. Gently press down with your knees while your hands push up (your hands produce resistance). Hold the press for a count of five. Repeat ten times. The "Tailor's Press" targets the inner thigh and gluteal muscles, making them better able to support the squatting position.

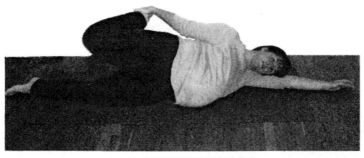

QUADRICEPS STRETCH

Lie on your left side. Rest your head on your outstretched arm. Bend your right leg and with your right hand, grab your foot, and pull up. You will feel a stretch through the front of your thigh (quadriceps muscles) and hip (hip flexors). Hold stretch for up to twenty seconds and then repeat on the other side. Your partner can help you with this stretch by holding your leg for you.

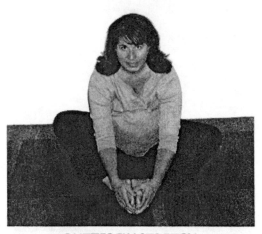

BUTTERFLY STRETCH

Sit on the floor and position legs so that the soles of your feet are touching. Pull your feet inward as close to your body as feels comfortable. Grab your feet with your hands. Keeping your back and spine straight, bend forward from your hips until you feel a stretch in your inner thighs. Hold stretch for up to twenty seconds. Butterfly stretches target inner thigh, hip, and gluteal muscles. Perform this stretch after you practice squatting.

ARM EXERCISES

These strengthening and stretching exercises target the arms and help prepare your body for carrying a newborn baby—and lugging around things like the car seat, stroller, and 48-pack cases of diapers! To do these exercises you can use light hand weights or soup cans.

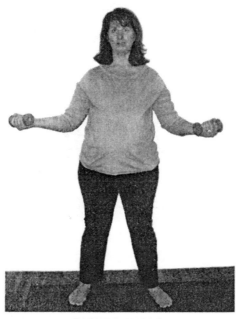

BICEPS CURLS

Stand with your feet shoulder-width apart, with your legs slightly bent, and your back flat. Hold a weight in each hand, with your elbows slightly bent. Slowly bend your arms, bringing your hands toward your shoulders. Exhale as you lower your arms back to their original position. Repeat 10 to 15 times.

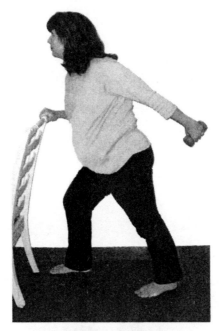

TRICEPS EXTENSIONS

Position a kitchen chair twelve to twenty-four inches in front of you. Hold a light hand weight or soup can in your left hand, and stand with feet hip-width apart, knees slightly bent. Take a small step forward with your right foot. Keep your back straight and bend forward from the hips until your head is in line with your right foot. Place your right hand on your right thigh or the chair for support. Bend your left arm into an L-shape so that the elbow is higher than your back. Without moving your elbow or upper arm, extend your lower arm backward, pause, and then slowly return your arm to the starting L-shaped position. Repeat 10 to 15 times on each side.

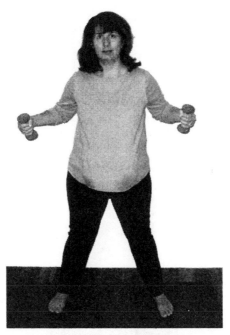

LATERAL RAISES

This exercise is good for your shoulders. Stand with feet shoulder-width apart. Your legs are slightly bent and your abdominal muscles tightened. Hold a weight or can of soup in each hand. Slightly bend your arms and bring your hands together so the weights touch. Using a slow, controlled movement, raise both arms to shoulder height. Lower back to original position. Inhale as your lift and exhale as you release. Repeat 10 to 15 times.

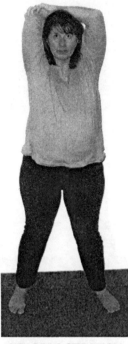

TRICEPS STRETCH

Stand with your feet shoulder-width apart, and your knees slightly bent. Tilt your pelvis. Use your left hand to pull your right elbow toward your head. You will feel a mild stretch in the back of your right arm. Hold stretch for up to twenty seconds. Repeat on left side.

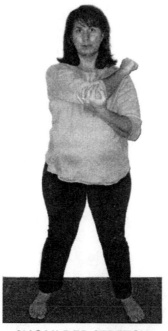

SHOULDER STRETCH

Stand or sit. Place your left hand on your right elbow and pull your right arm closer to your chest until you feel a stretch in your shoulder. Hold stretch for up to twenty seconds. Slowly release. Repeat by holding your left elbow with your right hand.

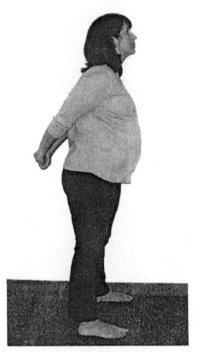

CHEST STRETCH

Stand with your feet shoulder-width apart. Check to make sure you have good posture. Clasp your hands behind the small of your back. Gently stretch your arms outward and down to feel a stretch in your chest and spine (your shoulders will be pulled back as you stretch, and it will feel like your chest is opening up). Hold the stretch for up to twenty seconds. Slowly release.

STRETCHING AND STRENGTHENING ESSENTIALS

- **Stay off your back.** After the 20th week of pregnancy, don't perform stretching and strengthening exercises while lying flat on your back. Exercising in this position allows your growing uterus to put too much pressure on the vena cava—the vein responsible for carrying blood from the lower body back to the heart. This can disrupt blood and oxygen flow to your baby and may cause you to feel faint or lightheaded.
- **Warm up.** Five to ten minutes of a light aerobic warm-up is a good way to prepare your muscles for stretching and strengthening. If you take a prenatal aerobics class, you will stretch just

after the warm-up portion of the workout and perform both stretching and strengthening exercises after the cooldown. You can mimic this routine when you exercise at home.

- **Keep breathing.** Breathe naturally while exercising. Holding your breath for prolonged periods of time may elevate blood pressure and reduce oxygen flow to your baby.

- **Avoid overstretching.** Pregnancy hormones and increasing pressure from your growing abdomen make your joints and tendons more vulnerable to injury during pregnancy. Overstretching may cause pulls, tears, and joint problems. If you feel pain when you stretch or if the tension in your muscles feels greater than before, you are probably overstretching. Stretch only to the point of mild tension and then release.

- **Keep it steady.** Reduce stress on your joints by avoiding jerky and bouncy movements while exercising. Focus on making all your movements flowing and smooth.

- **It shouldn't hurt.** Especially if you are new to working out, muscle fatigue is normal as you exercise muscles for the first time. However, "no pain, no gain" doesn't apply during pregnancy. Toning and stretching exercises should not cause pain or make you hurt. If they do, discontinue your workout and call your provider. See "Aerobic Exercise Dos and Don'ts" section for other warning signs to watch for during any physical activity.

Weekly Exercise Log

Tracking your daily exercise routine can give you a sense of accomplishment and purpose. It also serves more practical applications. If your muscles are extremely sore after working out you will know the activities to cut back on temporarily or eliminate. Bring your exercise log to prenatal appointments. Your provider determines how your fitness routine affects your pregnancy by monitoring your blood pressure, your weight gain, and your baby's heart rate. Being able to analyze your workout routine makes your provider better equipped to make suggestions for adjustments—and offer verbal affirmation for all your efforts to achieve a healthy pregnancy.

Here's how one sister successfully incorporated physical fitness into her pregnancy experience. You will see one week from her prenatal fitness routine. A sample exercise log for your own use follows.

Name: Lisa
Age: 26
Prepregnancy weight: 250
Prepregnancy exercise level: Sedentary

Exercise experience: I began exercising early in the second trimester. I started out by going on brief ten-minute walks a few times a week. Then I walked for fifteen minutes almost every day—and increased the pace and frequency of my workouts from there. After about three weeks of gradually building up, I could briskly walk for thirty minutes straight. I kept walking right up until my baby was born. Even though my pace slowed way down during the third trimester, if I could find enough bathrooms, my body was physically fit enough to walk for miles. I actually walked the mile or so to the hospital for one of my last prenatal appointments. Fortunately, I passed by the town library and enough restaurants to ensure plenty of potty breaks!

Exercising during pregnancy made me feel incredibly alive and healthy. I could sense my strength and endurance growing on an almost daily basis. Because my body became so accustomed to my daily workouts, it was easy to resume exercising after my baby was born. I'm now fitness walking up to three miles a day and am down thirty pounds from my prepregnancy weight!

LISA'S EXERCISE LOG

Week of ___ to ___	Sunday	Monday	Tuesday	Wednesday	Thursday	Friday	Saturday
Aerobic Activity Types/Minutes	Walked/20 mins	Walked/30 mins	Prenatal aerobics video/30 mins		Walked/30 mins	Swam/35 mins	Walked/40 mins
Back/Abs Strengthener/Reps	pelvic tilts/30×	belly breathing/30×	pelvic tilts/30×		child's pose/1 min double stars	extensions/20×	pelvic tilts/30×
Stretches	child's pose/1 min	child's pose/1 min	child's pose/1 min			child's pose/1 min	child's pose/1 min
Kegels Counts/Reps	3 seconds/20×	3 seconds/20×	3 seconds/25×		3 seconds/25×	3 seconds/30×	3 seconds/30×
Squats Strengthener/Reps	wall squats/5×	tailor press/10×	Wall squats/5×		chair squats/6×	wall squats/10×	chair squats/3×
Stretches	quads stretch	butterfly stretch	butterfly stretch		butterfly stretch	quads/stretch	(too sore for squats)
Arm Exercises Strengthener/Reps	biceps/10× triceps/10× lats/10×	lats/10×	lats/10×		lats/10×	lats/10×	biceps/10× triceps/10× lats/10×
Stretches	triceps chest and shoulder stretch	chest stretch	chest stretch		chest stretch	chest stretch	triceps chest and shoulder stretch
Fitness Notes	I'm finally getting the hang of kegels. Still not great at squatting	Always love how belly breathing seems to wake baby up and really get him kicking.	Laughed hysterically at e-mail jokes. No leaks! Kegels must be working!	Stayed late at work so I skipped exercise. Should have walked in the a.m.	I love how pregnancy made me finally start exercising. I feel great.	Shocked I could swim laps as long as I did. My hair is a wreck—buy swim cap.	Sharon came with me today. It's easier to walk longer when you have company.

SAMPLE EXERCISE LOG

Week of ___ to ___	Sunday	Monday	Tuesday	Wednesday	Thursday	Friday	Saturday
Aerobic Activity Types/ Minutes							
Back/Abs Strengthener/Reps Stretches							
Kegels Counts/Reps							
Squats Strengthener/Reps Stretches							
Arm Exercises Strengthener/Reps Stretches							
Fitness Notes							

Creating an Active Lifestyle

"I'm too busy to exercise" just didn't cut it anymore. After talking to my OB about all the good exercise could do for my plus-size pregnancy, I stopped making excuses and finally made physical activity a priority in my life. At first I was very embarrassed to go to the gym—like I didn't have the right to be there because of my weight. I told my OB about this and he recommended a prenatal water aerobics class at the local YMCA he had heard was excellent. My OB was right about the class—it was a wonderful introduction to working out. The instructor led us through a fun and challenging routine, told funny pregnancy stories, and taught me the basics of how to check heart rate and physical exertion. I got to know a lot of other women due around the same time—including many plus-size women.

A few of us who met in class are still working out together, even though our babies were born almost a year ago. Not only do I still take a water aerobics class three times a week, I even have a gym membership. Besides becoming a mother, becoming physically active was the biggest change I experienced as a result of my pregnancy.

—KRISTEN, age 27

IF YOU HAVE your own list of excuses for avoiding exercise, take time to compile another list—this one filled with tips for making physical activity a natural part of your everyday lifestyle. To help you reach your prenatal fitness goals, use the following suggestions and strategies to stay motivated and excited about your exercise routine:

- **Enlist your partner.** Exercise with your partner whenever possible. Your partner can provide moral support and motivation to stick with your workout. Taking a daily walk together is important "couple time" before the baby is born and is a positive step toward physical activity becoming a family habit. As you enter the third trimester, your partner can physically assist you with your stretching and strengthening exercises.
- **Take a prenatal exercise class.** Especially if you are pressed for time in your daily schedule, taking a prenatal exercise class is like one-stop shopping for your basic fitness needs. Prenatal exercise classes usually consist of a low-impact or water aerobics segment, plus stretching and toning exercises. Trained instructors lead class members through the entire routine, modeling proper posture and safe range of movement. You will know

exactly what to do and how long to do it for. Classes typically last only an hour. For women who don't have the time to construct their own fitness routine, a prenatal aerobics class might be the perfect fit.

The other benefit is, of course, bonding with other moms-to-be. Check out your hospital, YMCA, or community center for listings of prenatal exercise classes. Organizations offering exercise classes to expectant women require you to obtain your provider's written approval before you officially enroll.

- **Rest is important, too.** Listen to your body. As pregnancy progresses, especially in the latter months, you will probably receive strong signals from your body telling you to slow down and take it easy. Follow your instincts and rest when you need to. Don't force yourself to exercise if you are physically not up to it. Get a massage or listen to calming music. If you are relaxing in bed, regularly lift and rotate your ankles to maintain good circulation.

- **Exercise in the morning.** There are lots of good reasons to work out before noon: you are less tired, it's not as hot out, and exercising in the morning can rev your energy levels for the rest of the day. Try going for a brisk walk just after breakfast. Many YMCAs and health clubs are open as early as 6:00 a.m., enabling you to start your day by swimming laps or taking a low-impact aerobics class. For busy women, getting up a little earlier and exercising before work is an easy way to schedule physical activity into a hectic lifestyle.

- **Change your habits.** Even if you can't make it to the gym five nights a week, take simple steps to incorporate more activity into your everyday routine. Small changes can add up to make you stronger and more physically fit:

  - Don't drive if you can walk to your destination.
  - Hide your TV remote (or don't look for it the next time it's lost) and change channels the old-fashioned way.
  - Wash and dry the dishes by hand.
  - Take the stairs instead of the elevator.
  - Park farther out in the parking lot at work or the mall.
  - Hang laundry on a clothesline.
  - Use a manual-push lawn mower instead of a gas or electric version. Let your own body be the "horse power."

- **Keep it fresh.** One the quickest ways to lose interest in exercise is letting your fitness routine become boring. Prevent exercise monotony by taking steps to:

  - Vary your activities throughout the week. It's reassuring to have a routine, but doing the same exercises day after day for months may turn physical fitness into drudgery. Whether it's your weekly prenatal yoga class or swimming at the YMCA pool every Friday with your family, give yourself something different to look forward to.
  - Tired of walking by the same scenery day after day? Plan a weekend vacation or simple day trip to the beach to walk along the shoreline (walking in sand also gives your legs a better workout). Visit a big city and walk around the downtown shopping area. Many cities have "trails," mapped-out walks to lead tourists through the local historic districts. Check out if the nearby big city (or the one you live in) offers walking tours and become a tourist for the day.
  - Help others while you exercise by participating in local charity walks. Turn your prenatal fitness routine into the chance to join others in support of a good cause. Some events even supply portable toilets along the route—perfect for pregnant participants.

The best motivation might be to simply remind yourself what your hard work is for. As blood pressure readings hopefully remain within normal range, your weight gain continues at a slow and steady pace, and your baby's heartbeat is heard thumping away at all your prenatal checkups, know that exercise is playing no small role in your plus-size pregnancy's good health.

7

GESTATIONAL DIABETES

Steps to Success

The "up-side" to developing gestational diabetes? You can actually take steps to control the problem. This isn't one of those complications where all you are able to do is worry about whether or not it's going to grow worse. No matter how disappointed I was to encounter any problem with my pregnancy, it brought me great comfort to know I had the ability to keep my blood sugar levels within normal range.

—GINA, age 26

GESTATIONAL DIABETES IS a temporary form of high blood sugar that appears during pregnancy. Approximately 1 in 20 pregnant women will develop gestational diabetes, making it one of pregnancy's most common complications. Because entering pregnancy overweight or obese increases your chances for encountering this disorder, educating yourself about gestational diabetes is especially important for you as a plus-size woman.

This chapter serves as a springboard for you to discuss with your prenatal care provider your individual risk factors and the measures your provider will take to monitor your pregnancy for high blood sugar levels. If you are reading this chapter because you were just diagnosed with gestational diabetes, you will learn how you and your prenatal health-care team will work together to keep your pregnancy healthy. As

Gina and countless other sisters have learned, the "good news" about gestational diabetes is understanding that you have the power to ensure your health and protect your baby's well-being.

What Is Gestational Diabetes?

WHEN YOU HAVE gestational diabetes, your body is unable to properly use *glucose,* a simple sugar provided by the foods you eat. Glucose is the body's most basic form of energy, furnishing your cells with essential fuel. Fats and proteins break down into glucose, but carbohydrates in your diet most readily supply this necessary sugar. Every time you eat rice, cookies, fruit, bread, or other sweet or starchy foods, your digestive system converts the carbohydrates these foods contain into glucose.

As the food is digested, glucose enters the bloodstream. Your body responds to increased blood glucose ("blood sugar") levels by releasing insulin, a hormone produced in the pancreas. Certain cells, like muscle cells, need insulin in order to absorb glucose and use it as fuel. Insulin helps glucose leave the bloodstream and enter individual cells, enabling you to benefit from the energy the sugar provides.

While the exact cause of gestational diabetes is unknown, medical researchers believe hormones produced by the placenta interfere with the body's sensitivity to insulin. When you develop gestational diabetes, insulin is blocked from performing its vital work. Your pancreas still produces the hormone, but your cells begin to "resist" the insulin, greatly reducing the amount of glucose absorbed. As cells become more and more resistant, your body produces larger quantities of insulin. This can help for a short time, but insulin production soon cannot keep up with the ever-increasing demand. Without enough insulin to help glucose enter resistant cells, high levels of glucose pile up in the bloodstream.

Blood sugar levels typically spike after eating refined carbohydrates, mainly sugary foods and beverages that are quickly digested. When you are diabetic, your body simply cannot handle large amounts of rapidly produced glucose. When blood sugar levels in women with gestational diabetes are measured, even hours after consuming certain "trigger foods," the amount of glucose remaining in the blood is significantly higher than blood sugar levels found in women without gestational diabetes.

Most women who develop gestational diabetes do so between the 24th and 28th week of pregnancy, just as the placenta's hormone production begins to peak. In most cases, gestational diabetes disappears after the baby is born and the placenta is no longer present to cause insulin resistance.

Why Should I Care, if This Is Only Temporary?

GESTATIONAL DIABETES, LIKE all pregnancy complications, carries with it some health risks for both mother and baby. However, making a commitment to control blood sugar levels can dramatically reduce how likely you are to develop any further problems. The majority of women who take steps to keep their gestational diabetes in check go on to have successful pregnancies and healthy babies. Women with poorly controlled blood sugar levels put themselves and their babies at increased risk for encountering one or more of the following conditions:

- **Macrosomia:** For babies, the most common side effect of gestational diabetes is high birth weight. This is known in medical terms as *macrosomia*, which means a baby weighing more than approximately 10 pounds at birth. Your bloodstream is a pipeline to your growing baby, delivering nourishment through the placenta and umbilical cord. Too much glucose in your bloodstream means too much nourishment for your baby. Just like adults who eat too many sweets, your baby will store excess sugar as fat. If enough excess sugar needs to be stored as fat, the result is a baby with a high birth weight.

    High-birth-weight babies born to mothers with diabetes tend to accumulate fat in the shoulder area. This can make vaginal delivery much more difficult. In rare cases, high-birth-weight babies may suffer *shoulder dystocia*, or difficulty in delivering the shoulders of the baby once the head has emerged from the vagina. Also, women who give birth to high-birth-weight babies are more likely to deliver by cesarean section.

- **Hypoglycemia:** If you fail to control your gestational diabetes, your baby will produce large quantities of its own insulin to handle the high levels of sugar coming in from your bloodstream. When your baby is born and no longer needs all that extra insulin, your newborn's blood glucose can drop to very low levels. This is known as *hypoglycemia*. Most often, this low blood sugar responds to early feeding. In extreme cases, your newborn is given an infusion of glucose to keep blood sugar levels balanced.

- **Preeclampsia:** Women with gestational diabetes face an increased chance of developing preeclampsia. Preeclampsia is hypertension arising during pregnancy that is accompanied by protein in the urine and edema (swelling). Preeclampsia can pose many serious health problems for both mother and baby. Read chapter 4 for more information.

Risk Factors

ELENA, 30 POUNDS overweight when she conceived her first child, never developed gestational diabetes. Jessica, expecting her third child and 40 pounds above her ideal weight, did. Kathy, carrying 50 extra pounds and expecting baby number two, had normal blood sugar levels. Maria, Kathy's skinny friend, was not so lucky.

So who exactly gets gestational diabetes? Women of all shapes and sizes, and from many different backgrounds and experiences. The National Institute of Child Health and Human Development lists the following as key risk factors:

- **Family history of diabetes:** Your chances of developing gestational diabetes increase if a member of your immediate family has diabetes.
- **Overweight or obesity:** Women who are 20 percent or more above their ideal weight are more likely to develop gestational diabetes.
- **Ethnic group:** Hispanic, African-American, Native American, South or East Asian, Pacific Islander, and Native Australian women tend to have higher occurrences of gestational diabetes.
- **Personal health history:** Women who developed gestational diabetes in a past pregnancy, have given birth to a very large baby (weight above 9 pounds), or who have ever experienced a stillbirth, are all at greater risk for developing gestational diabetes during their current pregnancy.
- **Multiple-birth pregnancy:** Women pregnant with multiples are two to three times as likely to develop gestational diabetes.
- **Age:** Women over twenty-five years of age are statistically more likely to encounter high blood sugar levels during pregnancy.

Because many of these risk factors are so common (for example, most women in the U.S. are older than twenty-five when they become pregnant), prenatal care providers screen *all* women for gestational diabetes.

Are Plus-Size Women at Highest Risk?

Women who are overweight or obese do have higher rates of gestational diabetes than does the rest of the pregnant population, but this doesn't seem to tell the whole story. When looked at individually, many of these plus-size women also possess one or more additional risk factors (for instance, they may be overweight with a strong family history of diabetes, or obese and a member of a high-risk ethnic group). It appears that a combination of risk factors determines how likely you are to encounter this complication. Simply being overweight or obese does not guarantee you will develop gestational diabetes.

Bottom line? When discussing your pregnancy with your provider, don't skim over family-health background questions or omit personal information that makes you feel uncomfortable. Be honest about your own health history. This can only help you and your provider to more accurately monitor your pregnancy for diabetes.

Diagnosing Gestational Diabetes

To DETERMINE IF you have gestational diabetes, your provider evaluates how well your body metabolizes (absorbs) large amounts of glucose. Women are typically tested for gestational diabetes between the 24th and 28th week of pregnancy, the most likely time for high blood sugar levels to appear.

As described in chapter 4, the first step in the screening process is the one-hour glucose challenge test (GCT). If test results indicate blood sugar levels below 140 mg/dl (milligrams of glucose per deciliter of blood), it's unlikely you have gestational diabetes. Because pregnancy hormones often interfere to produce inaccurately high measurements, GCT results showing blood glucose levels above 140 mg/dl require further testing before confirming gestational diabetes.

The three-hour glucose tolerance test (GTT) truly determines whether or not you have gestational diabetes. Because you must fast for approximately ten hours before the test, the GTT is usually performed first thing in the morning. When you arrive for testing, the lab technician draws a blood sample to evaluate your fasting blood glucose levels. You then drink the same kind of sugary glucola beverage as during the one-hour screening (this one has twice as much sugar in it). Blood is drawn once an hour for three hours after drinking the glucola. When testing is complete, you may resume normal eating habits.

While awaiting your results, save your sanity by knowing in advance the notification process used by your provider. Are you contacted only if blood sugar levels are cause for concern? In how many days should you expect the results? What steps should you take if testing determines you do have gestational diabetes?

Gestational diabetes is diagnosed when two of the four blood draws from your GTT indicate higher than normal levels of glucose. Current guidelines define the cutoff for normal blood glucose levels as follows:

Fasting:	95 mg/dl
One hour:	180 mg/dl
Two hours:	155 mg/dl
Three hours:	140 mg/dl

If you *are* diagnosed with gestational diabetes, your prenatal care team will teach you exactly what you need to know in order to keep your blood sugar levels within normal range.

General guidelines for how women with gestational diabetes can keep their pregnancies healthy are described in the following sections.

Managing Your Gestational Diabetes

THE TREATMENT PLAN for gestational diabetes has one common theme: each step must be tailor fit to a woman's individual needs. Our advice is not meant to replace a customized strategy for controlling blood sugar levels. We offer a basic outline of how gestational diabetes is managed in *most* cases—a combination of diet, exercise, home blood glucose monitoring, and possible use of insulin injections. Members of the sisterhood whose stories we highlight each worked closely with her prenatal care team and the results speak for themselves.

What Do I Eat?

I remember it was early evening when my doctor called to tell me I had gestational diabetes. He arranged for me to meet with the practice's nutritionist the next morning. All that night, I was in a panic. I was scared to put anything in my mouth because I had no idea what I should be eating. I knew certain carbohydrates were bad if you had diabetes, but that was about it. I think I ended up eating peanut butter and cheese for dinner.

When I met with the nutritionist, it was a relief to get some real information. She told me exactly how many and what kinds of carbohydrates to eat over the course of the day, even giving me an exact number of carbohydrate grams to eat at every meal. I went home determined to make this new diet work. I cleared out all the sugary snack foods from our cupboards, made a grocery list, and restocked with diabetic-friendly choices. I created menus, read labels, checked portion sizes, and recorded my food intake on a daily basis.

Once I became informed about how to bring my blood sugar levels under control through healthy menu planning, the panic I had experienced that first night thankfully went away. I won't deny it, changing my eating habits on a dime was hard work, but so very worth it! My daughter was born a healthy seven pounds ten ounces.

—JACQUELINE, age 29

You are what you eat, and so is your blood sugar! For many women diagnosed with gestational diabetes, blood sugar levels are brought under control simply by eating a limited number of carbohydrates spread out over the course of many meals and snacks. Shortly after you are diagnosed with gestational diabetes, you will meet with a nutritionist to develop a "diabetic diet" custom-fit to your unique dietary needs as a pregnant woman. The following factors determine what menu plan is best for you:

- **Carbohydrate counts:** Your personalized diet includes the total number of carbohydrates you should eat each day. The American Diabetes Association currently recommends for women with gestational diabetes to consume 35 to 40 percent of calories from carbohydrates, and the rest of their calories from proteins and fats. Your nutritionist translates this percentage into a target number of carbohydrate grams to eat at each meal and snack. Because the body's insulin production is naturally at its lowest point in the morning, breakfast usually contains the smallest amount of carbohydrates.

  To help you make healthy food choices, your nutritionist will teach you the carbohydrate counts and serving sizes of most common foods (and how to read food labels for carbohydrate/sugar information). You will learn how to make meals and snacks that balance carbohydrate with proteins and fats. Eating carbohydrates in combination with protein and/or fat (such as peanut butter spread on whole grain crackers) slows down the rate at which carbohydrates break down into glucose and enter the bloodstream. Proteins and fats in food also leave you feeling more satisfied after eating.

(Note: Some nutritionists follow the "exchange" system formulated by the American Diabetes Association. This is just another easy way of menu planning and keeping track of carbohydrate intake.)

- **Carefully chosen carbohydrates:** Your nutritionist teaches you how to choose foods that help you maintain good control over your blood sugar levels. You will be instructed to avoid refined carbohydrates: sugar, processed grains, and high-fructose corn syrup. Foods and beverages such as regular soda, fruit juice, table sugar, honey, maple syrup, desserts made from refined flours, white bread, white rice, ice cream and sweetened frozen yogurt, and candy contain easily digested sugars that sharply raise blood sugar levels in most women with gestational diabetes.

  You don't need to avoid carbs altogether. You will be encouraged instead to eat those carbohydrates that are less likely to spike your blood sugar. These include high-fiber fruits and vegetables, whole-wheat breads, brown rice and other whole grains, and beans and legumes and their products (such as hummus and natural peanut butter). These carbohydrates digest at a slower rate than refined carbohydrates, meaning glucose is more gradually released into the bloodstream.

  Nutritionists sometimes use the phrase *glycemic index* when discussing how to choose carbohydrates for your diet plan. The glycemic index simply ranks foods from high to low based on how likely the food is to raise blood sugar levels. Refined carbohydrates—you guessed it—rank high on the glycemic index, whereas whole grains, beans, fruits, and vegetables tend to rank low. You will be urged to seek out low-glycemic-index foods.

- **Calories:** Your "diabetic diet" is *not a weight-loss diet*. Maintaining the weight-gain goals recommended by your OB is important to the overall health of your pregnancy. Gaining too much or too little weight can interfere with your baby's development and your ability to control your blood sugar. Your nutritionist will take into account your prepregnancy BMI and physical activity level to determine how many calories you should eat daily in order to stay on track for weight gain. You will receive suggestions on how to plan meals and snacks to meet your caloric requirements.

- **Consistency:** Your nutritionist might advise you to stick to a regular eating schedule, keeping the times you eat, and portion-size of your meals and snacks, roughly the same from day to day. Missing meals and snacks is not an option. Skipped carbohydrates added to the next meal or snack can overload your body with glucose and raise blood sugar levels.

- **Healthy options:** It's not easy to change eating habits overnight. Your nutritionist knows this and will provide you with plenty of suggestions for making nutritious, tasty meals and snacks, including recipes that take into consideration your personal food preferences.

Sample Menu

This one-day menu sample demonstrates how one sister's diet to control blood sugar levels translated into real-life eating.

Name: Holly

Diagnosed with gestational diabetes: 28 weeks

Prepregnancy BMI: 32

Activity level: moderate (Works as a teacher, on her feet for most of day. Goes to a prenatal swim class twice a week.)

Target daily carbohydrate grams: Approximately 250 g/day

Target calories for healthy weight gain: Approximately 2,100 calories/day

Breakfast: 6:30 a.m.—42 grams carbohydrates/ 340 calories

Menu	Carbohydrate Grams	Calories
1 egg	0 g	75
1 slice whole wheat toast	15 g	80
1 teaspoon butter	0 g	40
1 cup skim milk	12 g	85
1 small apple	15 g	60

continued

Snack: 9:30 a.m.—35 grams carbohydrates/280 calories

Menu	Carbohydrate Grams	Calories
6 crackers	15 g	80
1 tablespoon natural peanut butter	3 g	90
1 cup carrot sticks	5 g	25
1 cup skim milk	12 g	85

Lunch: 12:30 p.m.—55 grams carbohydrates/ 495 calories

Menu	Carbohydrate Grams	Calories
3 ounces skinless chicken (broiled)	0 g	140
1 teaspoon olive oil	0 g	45
2 tablespoons balsamic vinegar	6 g	30
2 cups mixed salad	10 g	50
6 ounces flavored whole-milk yogurt	24 g	170
½ cup strawberries	15 g	60

Snack: 3:30 p.m.—30 grams carbohydrates/ 255 calories

Menu	Carbohydrate Grams	Calories
1 small whole-grain muffin	15 g	80
1 tablespoon natural peanut butter	3 g	90
1 cup skim milk	12 g	85

Dinner: 6:00 p.m.—59 grams carbohydrates/ 515 calories

Menu	Carbohydrate Grams	Calories
1 turkey burger (3 ounces)	0 g	190
1 whole wheat kaiser roll	30 g	160
1 tablespoon catsup	4 g	15
1 cup mixed salad (put on burger)	5 g	25
1 teaspoon butter	0	40
½ cup cooked spinach	5 g	25
1 cup diced honeydew melon	15 g	60

Snack: 9:30 p.m.—30 grams carbohydrates/ 240 calories

Menu	Carbohydrate Grams	Calories
6 crackers	15 g	80
1 ounce cheese	0 g	100
½ cup strawberries	15g	60

Can I Really Make This Diet Work?

YOU HAVE MET with a nutritionist and constructed the perfect menu plan—now what? What happens when you open up the cupboards only to find your husband's stash of cookies? Can you avoid all the junk food lying around the break room at work? How will you handle that big sheet cake your mom already ordered for your baby shower? From the many sisters who have successfully followed a diabetic menu plan come the following tips and tactics for overcoming common obstacles to healthy eating:

- **Avoid "trigger foods."** If you notice a particular food makes your blood glucose levels spike, don't give it a second chance. Shrimp scampi, served over ¼ cup of spaghetti made from refined flour, might send your blood sugar skyrocketing. The same shrimp scampi served over ½ cup of brown rice or whole wheat spaghetti (a whole-grain carbohydrate), might keep blood sugar levels within normal range. Once you recognize your own "trigger foods," put them on the banned list until after your baby is born.
- **Beware hidden sugars.** If you are not already, become a label reader. Hidden sugars pop up where you least expect (bottled salad dressings are notoriously high in sugar). Once you become aware of how many sugars/carbohydrates are in certain foods, it becomes easier to make healthy choices. Instead of drowning your salad in your favorite dressing, possibly spiking your blood sugar, use a measuring spoon to measure out one serving. Or, simply switch to naturally low-carb olive oil and vinegar.
- **Avoid artificial sweeteners.** If sugary foods prove too difficult to completely give up, discuss with your nutritionist which artificial sweeteners, if any, are okay to use during pregnancy. The FDA recognizes aspartame (Nutrasweet) and sucralose (Splenda) as generally safe for most pregnant women, but even pregnancy-approved artificial sweeteners should be used sparingly—or not at all. Eating a slice of whole wheat toast spread with natural peanut butter is much more nutritious than eating an artificially sweetened candy bar. Your diet is carefully planned to control blood sugar levels AND provide proper nourishment for you and your growing baby. Always make the healthiest choice.

- **Plan in advance for handling celebrations.** Getting through holidays and special occasions such as birthdays and baby showers can be especially difficult when you have diabetes. Foods typically served at family gatherings (soda, punch, cake, cookies, white bread, etc.) are the foods you most need to avoid. How do you make it through all the festivities without doing major damage to your blood sugar control?

  Be honest with the party giver about your situation. Offer to make some of the food for the party yourself and prepare healthy alternatives less likely to raise blood sugar levels (cut raw vegetables with a yogurt dip, cubed cheese, whole wheat rolls, bran muffins, fresh fruit, nuts, etc.). Chances are, you are not the only one who is watching what they eat and these choices will be greatly appreciated.

  If you just don't think a celebration like a baby shower or birthday is the same without a cake, most bakeries do sell artificially sweetened versions. Ask to see the ingredient list before placing your order and then check with your nutritionist or provider to make sure the artificial sweetener used by the bakery is safe.

- **Prepare nutritious foods for work.** If your workplace overflows with sugary snacks, from the bowl of mini candy bars on the secretary's desk to the leftover birthday cake in the break room, go into counterattack mode. It's easier to avoid workplace temptation when you are not hungry. Be prepared by making your own lunch and snacks the night before. Pack appetizing foods you know will leave you satisfied. To really make a statement, bring enough of your own "goodies" for others to share. Let your co-workers rave over your homemade hummus dip with fresh cut veggies!

- **Dine out wisely.** Going out to dinner can still be an enjoyable part of your life. Just follow a few sensible modifications. Ask for a list of ingredients and their carbohydrate count before ordering (most restaurants have nutritional information readily available). Skip the soda and order ice water with lemon instead. Ask for substitutions whenever needed—trade white bread for whole wheat, french fries for veggies, etc. Don't even open the dessert menu! Finish off your meal by ordering a fresh fruit cup.

- **Enlist your loved ones.** Explain to your family why you sticking to this diet is so important. Give specific suggestions for how loved ones can help you succeed. Plan meals, go grocery shopping, and cook together. If you need junk food to be totally banned from the house, be up front about this and provide plenty of tasty and nutritious snack alternatives. Educate your family about gestational diabetes. Knowing how to choose healthy foods and measure portion sizes are good skills for anyone in the family to have.

- **Gather recipes.** Go online and find creative ways to "spend" your carbs over the course of your day. There are numerous Web sites dedicated to providing easy and delicious recipes for people following diabetic meal plans. See Resources for more information.

- **Seek support.** Most hospitals and many community centers have support groups for people with diabetes. These groups can be a source for information, assistance, and practical day-to-day strategies. Contact your hospital or look in the community health-events section of your local newspaper to see what kinds of support groups are available, and if there is one specifically for women with gestational diabetes. Many pregnancy and diabetes-related Web sites have message boards devoted to gestational diabetes. Connecting with other women in the same situation can be a powerful tool for coping with this complication.

- **Enjoy your food:** Create meals and snacks to both tantalize your taste buds and keep your blood sugar under control. Choose foods full of flavor: an omelet bursting with sun-sweet orange and yellow bell peppers; tart Granny Smith apple slices spread with salty and nutty natural peanut butter; a mile-high sandwich of turkey, tomato, cheese, sprouts, and tangy mustard served between two crunchy slices of whole wheat toast. With every bite of nutritious, carbohydrate-correct food, rejoice in knowing you are doing the very best for both you and your baby. Bon appétit!

Exercise

I walked around the track behind the local middle school, totaling at least two miles a day. Not only were my blood sugar levels excellent, I went from feeling really down and stressed out about the diabetes to feeling like I was in the best shape of my entire life. I now know gestational diabetes was the wake-up call I needed to pay more attention to my body's health.

—RENÉE, age 30

EXERCISE PROVIDES A wealth of benefits for women with gestational diabetes. Increased physical activity helps relieve stress and anxiety, strengthens muscles, improves cardiovascular fitness, and most important, helps keep blood glucose levels within normal range. When you exercise, cells become less resistant to insulin and more willing to absorb the glucose in your bloodstream. Something as simple as taking a brisk twenty-minute walk after eating has been shown effective in lowering blood glucose levels in women with gestational diabetes.

Always check with your provider to make sure physical activity is safe for your pregnancy. Some exercise suggestions from the many sisters who have walked briskly in your sneakers include:

- **Start small.** If you have never exercised, or have not exercised in a few years, start by taking a leisurely stroll through the neighborhood. Build up from there until your leisurely stroll becomes a twenty-minute power walk.
- **Exercise early and often.** Exercise after breakfast to help with sluggish morning insulin levels. At work, walk briskly around the building or around the block before returning from your lunch break. Walking in the evening brings down after-dinner glucose levels and even improves your fasting levels for the following morning.
- **Mall walk.** People around the country make use of their local mall as the perfect workout area. Malls are climate-controlled, so no need to worry about rain, snow, or heat. Stop by the mall's customer service desk to see what programs they offer for "mall walkers," or simply strap on your sneakers and get ready for some brisk window-shopping.
- **Add variety.** Although going for a quick walk is probably the easiest and most convenient way to work in postmeal exercise, other forms of physical activity will also help you control blood glucose levels. Swimming or participating in a low-impact aerobics class are excellent exercises, and are gentle on your pregnant body. Contact your local YMCA or hospital outreach center to find out what prenatal exercise classes are available in your area.

    If your provider advises you to refrain from exercise that engages the lower half of your body, you can still get a very good workout just from using your arms. Grab some hand weights and lift your arms over your head, then lower them back to your sides. Briskly repeat these basic arm-lifts for twenty minutes.

You are working out hard enough if you feel slightly out of breath. As you do this, play your favorite music, or watch TV to make the time go by faster.

No matter what type of physical activity you take part in, stop exercising and rest if you experience fatigue, dizziness, pain, or discomfort. Call your provider if symptoms persist. For more exercise suggestions, see chapter 6, "Prenatal Exercise."

Blood Glucose Monitoring

HOME BLOOD GLUCOSE monitoring is a simple task to quickly determine how well your gestational diabetes management plan is working. An expert from your provider's office (nurse practitioner, nutritionist, diabetes educator, or your provider) will show you how to easily track your blood glucose levels.

Diabetic-testing technology continues to improve, but the basics remain the same. A small handheld device called a *glucometer* is loaded with a diabetes-testing strip. Obtained by pricking one of your fingers with a tiny lancet, a small drop of blood is placed on the testing strip. In about twenty seconds (or only a few seconds on some newer models), a number appears on the glucometer screen. The number represents how many milligrams of glucose are present in each deciliter of blood (mg/dl).

Most women are instructed to measure blood glucose levels four times a day: upon waking (fasting blood glucose) and then two hours after each meal. Fasting blood glucose levels give an overall picture of how well your body is coping with gestational diabetes. Postmeal readings measure your body's ability to tolerate carbohydrates in your foods.

All blood glucose testing results are recorded in a chart and frequently submitted to your provider for review.

Date	Insulin Dose / Time	Fasting Level	Postbreakfast Level	Postlunch Level	Postdinner Level	Notes

SAMPLE BLOOD GLUCOSE TESTING RECORD

If your management plan to control gestational diabetes is working, your blood glucose levels should be the same as a woman without gestational diabetes. According to current standards, normal blood glucose ranges are:

Fasting: 60 mg/dl to 105 mg/dl
Before meal: 60 mg/dl to 95 mg/dl
1 hour after meal: 140 mg/dl or less
2 hours after meal: 120 mg/dl or less

Glucose Testing Tips

If incorporating glucose testing into your already hectic existence seems like an overwhelming task, use the following strategies to help make monitoring blood sugar levels an effortless part of your everyday routine:

- **Finger factor.** Pricking your fingers several times a day is probably not your idea of fun. Obtaining a blood drop can be made much less bothersome if you prick the side of your finger, rather than the finger pad. Finger pads are full of nerves and provide us with our sense of touch. Place your index finger on your thumb and then place your middle finger on top of your index finger. The side of the index finger showing between the other two contains fewer nerves and is much less sensitive (the same is true for all your fingers). Alternate fingers with each test to give your digits a chance to heal between prickings. To reduce the chance for infection, swab each finger with an alcohol-soaked cotton ball (or wipe) and *always* use a new lancet.
- **Replenish supplies.** Most women with gestational diabetes need to test blood sugar levels several times throughout the day. Be sure to have a constant supply of testing strips and lancets available, and an extra set of batteries for your glucometer. Because monitoring gestational diabetes is now part of your prenatal care, insurance companies will generally cover costs for all or most supplies.
- **Stay organized.** Place all supplies in a plastic container and keep it in a designated location out of reach of any children. Bring testing supplies along when you are on the road. Most glucometer models come in a compact carrying case with enough room for a few testing strips and lancets. For extended trips away from home, simply pack your plastic container.
- **Monitor at your workplace.** Don't let a busy workday get in the way of your glucose monitoring. From start to finish, diabetic testing takes less time than the average bathroom break. and you can easily do it there if you feel self-conscious about using the glucometer in front of others. Check into whether your insurance company will cover a second glucometer and additional supplies to use at work. This reduces the chance that you might forget your supplies and miss scheduled testing

times. Even if you end up paying out of pocket, a basic model retails for under $100. Your provider's office might be able to loan you an extra glucometer until your maternity leave begins. Ask if the practice has such a policy.

- **Time yourself.** For accurate results, take blood glucose measurements at the correct time. If you are supposed to test at two hours after eating, but end up testing three hours later with a blood glucose reading of 114 mg/dl, you will never know if at two hours you were under 120 md/dl or not. To remind yourself when to measure, set an alarm clock or timer. Even cell phones have an alarm function that can be pressed into service.

How Are the Test Results Used?

You will communicate your blood glucose testing results to your prenatal care team on a frequent basis (perhaps twice a week). Glucose levels are scrutinized for any high numbers, noting what time of day and how often higher-than-normal glucose levels are detected. Your care team also compares results from week to week to see if glucose levels show any pattern of gradually creeping higher.

When readings are cause for concern, several steps may be taken. You might need to return to your nutritionist to fine-tune your meal plan and carefully look over your food choices. Sometimes obtaining normal postmeal blood glucose levels may be as simple as exchanging an overlooked white-flour hamburger roll for a healthier whole wheat pita. You may be advised to increase your activity level after meals to see if more exercise will bring your glucose levels under control.

Blood glucose levels sometimes remain high, despite your best efforts. If blood glucose monitoring shows gestational diabetes has progressed beyond what diet and exercise alone can handle, insulin injections will be required to bring blood sugar levels within normal range.

Insulin

Change my diet? No problem. Exercise after meals? I plugged in my treadmill and began walking. Only problem? Diet and exercise just weren't doing the trick when it came to keeping my blood glucose levels in check. After four days straight of high fasting levels (110 mg/dl), my OB told me I would need to control my diabetes by injecting insulin. I met with the nutritionist again. This time, instead of talking about food, she showed me all the steps for injecting insulin. As the nutritionist helped me

*practice an insulin injection using an orange, I just kept thinking, will I really be able
to do this to myself for the two months left until my due date?*

*That night I did everything the nutritionist said to do and—as she promised—
injecting insulin was a quick and painless process. However simple injecting
insulin turned out to be, I still wasn't crazy about the idea. What finally boosted
my morale was taking my fasting blood sugar the next morning and seeing my
reading finally fall within normal range. That's when it hit me, injecting insulin
might not be anyone's idea of fun, but when you need it, it works. I suddenly felt
more relaxed than I had been since learning I had gestational diabetes. I was overcome with a sense that everything was going to be just fine.*

—LISA, age 28

When normal blood glucose levels are not achieved through diet and
exercise alone, your OB will prescribe insulin injections. After working hard to make diet and exercise modifications, being told you must
inject insulin can bring on feelings of frustration or even failure. Look
beyond your immediate reaction. Focus on how insulin is one more step
toward a successful pregnancy and a healthy baby.

Medical studies demonstrate that babies born to plus-size women
who use insulin during pregnancy have lower rates of macrosomia (high
birth weight) than babies born to plus-size women who don't even have
gestational diabetes. Injecting insulin has no negative side effects for
your developing baby. In fact, it's just the opposite. Although there are
many glucose-lowering agents on the market for people with Type II
diabetes, most of these medications are generally not used during
pregnancy.

Insulin used to control gestational diabetes comes in two varieties:
NPH (*intermediate-acting insulin*), and Humalog (*fast-acting insulin*).
You may be required to use one or both types of insulin.

- **NPH:** When blood glucose monitoring indicates fasting blood
  sugar levels are too high, NPH is generally prescribed. High
  fasting numbers are linked to glucose production by the liver.
  Your liver is your reserve fuel tank, storing glucose (in the
  form of glycogen) and then releasing it back into the bloodstream as your body signals for additional energy. The liver is
  often called upon to release glucose stores at night, when several hours have passed since your last meal.

  When your blood sugar levels are high first thing in the
  morning, it means your body's own insulin cannot handle this

extra glucose released at night. To bring levels under control, you will inject a prescribed amount of NPH at bedtime. NPH gradually enters your system, ready to help whenever liver-produced glucose is released in your body.

- **Humalog:** When high numbers constantly pop up after meals (above 120 mg/dl two hours postmeal), fast-acting Humalog insulin helps bring glucose levels back within the normal range. Humalog is injected just before eating, making it immediately available to help cells absorb glucose produced from the foods in your meal. Depending on your insulin needs, you may need to inject Humalog before one, two, or all of your daily meals.

Your provider will determine the correct amount of insulin needed to normalize your blood glucose levels. Because resistance to insulin generally increases as pregnancy progresses, this amount may rise as the weeks go by. Your care team will watch closely to see how your blood glucose levels respond to insulin use. Maintain a careful record of your insulin dose amount, and the times it is administered, alongside your blood glucose testing information, so that you can keep your provider up to date.

Administering Insulin

Injecting insulin is a relatively easy maneuver. Your nutritionist (or a diabetes educator), will show you how to load a hypodermic needle and where on your body to inject the insulin (upper arms and thighs are good sites). Some helpful tips for making this entire process simple and quick include:

- **Establish a routine.** Find a place in your house or at work that is private and free from distraction. Give yourself enough time to swab your arm or thigh with an alcohol wipe, correctly measure the dosage, inject the insulin, and safely discard used supplies.
- **Take care of your supplies.** Insulin must be stored according to the label's instructions. If you need to inject insulin while at work, ask your pharmacist to split your insulin prescription between two bottles. Leave one bottle at home, and use the other one while at your job. Keep hypodermic needles out of children's reach. *Always* use a new needle for each dose. Dispose of each used needle as described below.

- **Get help.** If you are squeamish about needles, enlist a friend or your partner to assist you. If this is not possible, you must be up front with your care team about your nervousness. They can practice with you until you are comfortable giving injections. Don't allow fear to get in the way of gaining control over gestational diabetes. Focus on the good insulin is doing for the well-being of both you and your baby.
- **Dispose of your needles properly.** Technically hazardous medical waste, used hypodermic needles must be disposed of in a safe and sanitary way. An empty, well-labeled laundry detergent jug is a good place to put used needles because the thick plastic prevents the needles from poking through. Check with your sanitation department about disposal regulations in your area. You might need to mark "medical waste" on the containers before you throw them away. Ask your nutritionist or diabetes educator for more information about safely discarding used supplies.
- **Watch for symptoms of hypoglycemia.** Sometimes insulin injections cause blood sugar levels to fall too low. Hypoglycemia (low blood sugar) has a number of recognizable symptoms: dizziness, lightheadedness, or even fainting. If you feel any of these symptoms coming on, you need to immediately eat a small amount of easily digested sugar. This will help to quickly raise your blood sugar levels. Drinking some orange juice, sucking on a piece of hard candy, or eating a cookie can help. Your nutritionist can give you more specifics about what to do if you experience low blood sugar.

Optional Tests

IN ADDITION TO blood glucose monitoring, your provider may decide a few more steps are necessary to make sure you and your baby are doing just fine. Some of these optional testing choices include:

- **Ultrasounds:** Ultrasounds supply vital information about your baby's growth and development, providing a snapshot of life in the womb. Your provider may use ultrasound during the last few weeks of pregnancy to monitor for possible fetal macrosomia. This information helps anticipate possible delivery concerns.

- **Nonstress tests:** If your gestational diabetes is treated with insulin, your provider may want you to undergo a weekly non-stress test (NST) starting around the 32nd–34th week of pregnancy. For women who manage their gestational diabetes through diet and exercise, your provider might administer a NST closer to your due date. This simple, noninvasive procedure is performed at your provider's office and requires no special preparation. The NST evaluates your baby's general well-being by measuring how the fetal heart responds when your baby moves.

  To perform an NST, a fetal heart monitor (Doppler ultrasound) is attached to your abdomen with a belt. A printer connected to the monitor prints out a fetal heart rate tracing for your baby. You push a button (also connected to the monitor) each time you feel the baby move, and this makes a mark on the tracing. Your provider then analyzes the printout, looking for your marks to correspond with increases in fetal heart rate. When your baby moves, its heart rate usually increases.

  Sometimes your baby is sleeping when you go in for the NST. If this is the case, you might be given something to eat or drink to help your baby wake up and start moving. If tests results show a "nonreactive" strip, meaning the baby did not move (despite various methods) or if the heart rate did not respond when there was movement, this *might* be a sign your baby is in distress. In more than 75 percent of nonreactive NST results, further testing proves the baby is just fine.

- **Kick counts:** In addition to nonstress tests performed in the office, your OB may ask you to do kick counts at home. All you need to do is sit still or lie quietly and record how many times you feel your baby move during a certain amount of time (your provider will give you specifics about how long to count for). Again, this simple procedure can provide reassurance about your baby's health and general well-being. Contact your provider's office if the kick count did not meet the minimum number of movements.

Childbirth and Beyond

MOST WOMEN WITH gestational diabetes who successfully control their blood glucose levels go on to experience perfectly normal vaginal deliveries. When looked at as a group, however, women with gestational diabetes are at higher risk for delivering their babies by cesarean section than are women without diabetes. Cesarean section is often considered when other complications arise.

Women with gestational diabetes are also more likely to have their labors induced. Some providers believe that delivering a baby a week or two before the estimated due date can reduce the likelihood of complications. The decision to induce is based on many variables. If your blood sugar levels are controlled and signs point to a healthy baby, there is probably no reason to induce labor.

Discuss your concerns about labor and delivery with your provider well in advance of your due date. For more about what plus-size women can expect during childbirth, please see chapter 9, "Labor and Delivery."

Postpartum

Gestational diabetes ends when the hormones in the placenta are no longer present to interfere with your body's sensitivity to insulin. Once the baby is born and the placenta delivered, blood sugar levels return to normal for almost all women who had gestational diabetes. To make sure your blood glucose levels are within normal range, you will need to report back to the lab about six weeks after delivery and have one more glucose tolerance test (this one may only last for two hours instead of three). For a small group of women (2 to 3 percent), blood glucose levels remain elevated. These women are diagnosed with Type II diabetes and require further care.

Because you experienced gestational diabetes during pregnancy, you are at increased risk for developing Type II diabetes later in life. According to the American Diabetes Association, you should have your blood sugar levels checked a minimum of once every three years. Fifty percent of women who experience gestational diabetes develop Type II diabetes within twenty-eight years of delivery.

The Future

When I look back at what I ate when I had gestational diabetes, it's easy to see how the diabetic diet is simply excellent nutrition. Even after my daughter was born and my blood sugar levels returned to normal, I'm proud to say I didn't go back to my old eating habits. The sugary foods and white bread are gone, hopefully forever.

—LISA, age 28

Maternity Clothes

In an attempt to camouflage my weight problem, my basic prepregnancy wardrobe consisted mainly of loose, baggy clothes. The only accommodation I needed to make for a bulging pregnant belly was to reach further back in the closet for my baggiest pairs of pants. Although I saved money by not buying maternity clothes, my partially obscured pregnant silhouette caused some people a lot of confusion. When I ran into old acquaintances and causally mentioned my impending due date, I became so accustomed to seeing the looks of surprise and disbelief that I stopped talking about my pregnancy with anyone except those closest to me. I was ready to scream the next time someone exclaimed, "You're pregnant? I had no idea!"

I told my mother how frustrated I was at what seemed like the entire world's inability to notice my pregnancy. A few days later, a package arrived in the mail. An early birthday present, as her enclosed note read, my mother had sent me several maternity shirts, all in my size. I put one on and looked in the mirror. It was the first time in years I had worn such a tailored, fitted shirt. I was stunned at how beautifully pregnant I looked.

I wore the shirt to work the next day and people were suddenly holding open doors, carrying things for me, complimenting me on my pregnant glow. While I liked finally getting recognition from others, that's not what mattered most. What truly made me happy was feeling more confident and pleased about my own appearance. Liberated from the usual assortment of shapeless shirts and oversized sweaters, I proudly showed off my pregnant body.

—CHRISTINE, age 26

MATERNITY CLOTHES ARE designed to accommodate a growing belly in comfort and style, but as Christine and many other plus-size women report, wearing maternity clothes also provides a much-needed body image boost. Some sisters might not "show" until the last few months of pregnancy while others pop out of their clothes well before the second trimester begins. No matter when you outgrow your regular wardrobe, all big, beautiful, and pregnant women can follow one simple rule when it comes to maternity fashions: choose clothing that makes you look as radiant and happy on the outside as you feel on the inside.

Finding trendy plus-size maternity clothes is much easier than in years past. Due to popular demand, several department and clothing store chains now stock sizes up to 3X, either in-store or through Internet/catalog sales. Some online-only maternity stores offer sizes up to 6X. (See Resources for sister-recommended plus-size maternity retailers.)

Shopping opportunities abound for the big, beautiful, and pregnant population but be forewarned: maternity clothes are often pretty pricey. Because you wear maternity clothes for such a short period of time, consider the following alternatives before hitting the mall or logging onto the Internet.

- **Buy gently worn.** Stretch your buying power by scouting out thrift or consignment shops, garage sales, and Web sites such as eBay for used plus-size maternity clothes at bargain prices. Because maternity clothes are worn for only a few months (or less), used clothing is often found in like-new condition. After your baby is born, consider donating or consigning your own gently worn maternity clothes.
- **Call on the sisterhood.** Plus-size women who blazed the pregnancy trail before you will probably be more than willing to let you borrow from their own stash of maternity clothes. Be thankful you know such generous women and some day return the favor to another sister-in-need!
- **Create a pregnant silhouette.** Buying regular plus-size clothes a size or two larger than what you normally wear is an easy and cheap alternative to a new maternity wardrobe. Roomy T-shirts and elastic-waist pants a size larger than normal might fit right through the third trimester. However, as Christine experienced, the drawback to this method of dressing is the tendency for oversize shirts to hide—rather than showcase—your growing belly. Even if you can't sew, you can slightly alter nonmaternity clothes to create a more "pregnant" silhouette. Use the following tricks to readily transform the tops you already own into custom-tailored maternity separates:

    - *Maternity clip:* Constructed from a short piece of elastic with suspender clips at either end, a maternity clip attaches to the back of any type of shirt (placed on the outside of the shirt—usually just below your braline). The clip gives you a more defined maternity shape because it pulls your shirt tighter under your bust while allowing the bottom half of the shirt to flare out around your belly. You can buy maternity clips at maternity clothing stores— clips often come in a variety of colors and styles. Another option is to shop the children's department. Maternity clips are identical to the clips sold to attach children's mittens to a winter coat. Mitten clips sell for only a few dollars—and you get two per package!

◆ No-sew maternity T-shirt: Extra roomy T-shirts are easily altered into fashionable maternity tops. Put on your favorite loose-fitting T-shirt and face a mirror where you can see yourself from at least the waist up. Just below the center of your bust line, create a front pleat by making two folds about an inch or two apart. Check your reflection to make sure the pleat is centered and the folds straight. Adjust as necessary. Hold the pleat in place by pinning a pretty brooch right where the folds begin. Your T-shirt now "poufs out" just below the bust, providing the look of a maternity T-shirt at a fraction of the cost.

■ **Celebrate in style!** Dressier outfits are often the most expensive and difficult to find of all plus-size maternity clothes. Look your best for special occasions by improvising with non-maternity dresses and separates. When you need more formal attire, wear dresses designed with an empire waistline, one that starts at or just below the bust and leaves plenty of room for your pregnant belly. Emphasize your expectant silhouette by sewing a one-inch-thick ribbon along the waist seamline of your dress (use basting stitches in thread the same shade as the ribbon).

Feel more comfortable wearing pants to your special occasion? Choose roomy pants with an elastic waist. Top with a silky shirt designed in a "baby doll," "trapeze," or "swing" style (a few sizes larger than what you wore prepregnancy might fit best depending on how far along you are). Use a maternity clip or create a front pleat as described above to give your dressy outfit a more fitted shape.

■ **Splurge at least once or twice.** If your budget allows, buy one or two articles of maternity clothing that make you look as beautiful as you feel. If you end up splurging on only one maternity shirt, keep your look fresh by pairing your top with a shawl one day and an unbuttoned cardigan sweater or blazer the next. Extend your wardrobe by mixing and matching a few new maternity pieces with nonmaternity separates that still fit.

Whatever you end up wearing during pregnancy, pick comfortable clothes that express your personal style. Love bright colors? Like wild prints? Wear them. Tie a pretty scarf in your hair or sparkle from head to toe with your favorite jewelry. Take time to look like the hip mama-to-be you truly are!

A NOTE ABOUT PLUS-SIZE BELLIES . . .

EVERY PLUS-SIZE woman is unique—and so is her pregnant belly. When will you begin to show? Will you develop a perfect round orb of a belly? The answers to these questions vary greatly among plus-size women. Generally speaking, if you have given birth before or if you are currently pregnant with multiples, you may notice your belly begin to swell as early as the end of the first or beginning of the second trimester. Pregnant for the first time? A noticeably rounder pregnant belly may start to show sometime during your fifth month. An apple-shaped woman who carried excess weight in her stomach area prepregnancy may notice this weight shifts downward as her pregnant belly expands. Larger women who gain a minimal amount of weight during pregnancy may find themselves starting to show much later than women with higher weight-gain goals.

Always remember, no matter when your belly begins to change or what shape it takes, your pregnant belly is beautiful because of what's on the inside—a busily growing baby!

Celebrate Your Experience

My partner found some directions on the Internet for making a plaster belly cast. Neither of us is very crafty but it seemed like all those women on the cable networks' having-a-baby shows were always making these, so one quiet weekend before my due date we decided to give it a try. As the mold dried, I felt giddy by how perfectly pregnant my belly's plaster contour looked. Two years later, my belly cast still hangs prominently on our living room wall as a permanent reminder of my beautiful pregnant body.

—VIV, age 28

EVERY PREGNANT WOMAN deserves to feel good about herself. Need creative inspiration for turning your pregnancy into a celebration? Try some of the following sister-tested, sister-approved ideas to help you fill these nine months with happiness and joy:

- **Make a belly cast.** You and your partner can forever capture your body's amazing transformation by creating a belly cast, a three-dimensional mold formed by layering strips of plaster gauze across your pregnant belly. Belly casting kits are readily available, or simply visit your local craft store and buy seven or eight rolls of plaster gauze bandages, gesso (plaster paint to stiffen and stabilize the finished mold), extra-fine sandpaper, and paints to decorate the cast (optional). Double the amount of plaster gauze bandages if you plan to include your arms, thighs, and upper torso above your breasts. Other supplies you will need are: a drop cloth, scissors, two pencils, a clean bucket, and petroleum jelly.

  This project is best done a few weeks before your due date when your belly has reached peak roundness. Make your cast in a room with good ventilation and a comfortable place for you to sit. Prepare your workspace by spreading a drop cloth on the floor. Cut the plaster bandages into strips approximately 6, 10, and 12 inches long. Fill the bucket with lukewarm water.

  Generously coat with petroleum jelly the parts of your body you want to cast (belly, breasts, and possibly arms). The petroleum jelly allows the plaster gauze to more easily pull away from your body as it dries. Your partner should help with this task to make sure you don't miss any spots. If needed, use cotton padding to cover armpit, belly, or pubic hair.

  Once the chosen area is protected by petroleum jelly, strike a pose. An easy way to achieve a full, round shape is to sit on the edge of a chair with your hands clasped underneath your belly. Lying down will flatten out your pregnant shape and is not recommended.

  To begin casting, your partner dips a plaster gauze strip in the water bucket. The strip should be held taut so it doesn't fold or twist. Your partner lifts the strip from the bucket and squeezes away excess water by running it between two pencils held tightly together. Strip by strip, your partner starts applying the gauze to your body, overlapping and varying direction for a stronger cast. Your partner must work fast because the plaster sets quickly. After about twenty minutes, you will start to see the cast pull away from your body.

Once all the strips are applied, wait about five minutes before carefully removing the cast from your body (you may need to wiggle a bit to help the cast off). It will take about 48 hours for the mold to completely harden. You can strengthen the cast by painting it with gesso. Allow the gesso to dry and then smooth out the shape by sanding it with extra-fine sandpaper. Paint and decorate your cast with whatever design seems right. Some women choose abstract shapes and swirls, whereas others depict personally symbolic objects, scenes, or meaningful words and poems. Many leave it blank and let the shape speak for itself. As Viv chose to do, give this life-size tribute to your radiant pregnant shape a permanent place of honor in your home.

- **Become a work of art.** Belly painting is another fun, creative way to celebrate your pregnant body. With your belly as the canvas, let your partner, friends, or your other children transform your belly into anything from a smiling jack-o'-lantern to a multicolored Easter egg, fish tank, or snow globe. Use water-based nontoxic face paints for best results (test a small patch of skin first to make sure paints are nonirritating). Belly painting is a temporary art form, so remember to take lots of pictures!

- **Pamper yourself.** Honor your pregnant body by lavishly pampering it. Rub your belly with cocoa butter or apricot oil to help soften and soothe itchy skin (unfortunately, moisturizing your belly probably won't prevent stretch marks—though it doesn't hurt to try!). Take long bubble baths and giggle when you see your belly sticking up out of the water (avoid overheating while in the tub by making sure bath water is comfortably warm and not hot). Deep-condition your hair to make that pregnant mane even more thick and lustrous. Soak your tired, swollen feet in a bucket of cool water. Add a cup of Epsom salts for extra foot-soothing power. Achy legs? Have your partner massage your legs using upward strokes to improve circulation (and then instruct your partner to massage your aching back!). For a full day of nothing but pampering, check out which spas in your area cater to pregnant women.

- **Tell your own story.** Visually record your pregnancy by making a pregnancy scrapbook. You can invest in all the latest scrapbooking supplies, but a simple three-ring binder filled with inexpensive decorative paper is all you need to start transforming special photographs and little bits and pieces of pregnancy memorabilia into the unique story of your own experience. Thumb through scrapbooking magazines for inspiring design ideas. As Sarah found out, a meaningful—and easy—project is to regularly take pictures of your growing belly.

- **Celebrate yourself!** While it's exciting to constantly think about what life will be like after your baby arrives, indulge all those passions you might not have time for once you begin taking care of a newborn. Enroll in a college course and study a topic you have always found fascinating. Read novels and watch movies that have nothing to do with pregnancy or parenthood. See a play. Paint a self-portrait. Learn a foreign language. Go out for a fun night of dancing. Get away for the weekend with your girlfriends or jet off with your partner to your favorite vacation spot (most women can safely fly until the 36th week of pregnancy, but always run your travel plans by your provider first).

However you choose to celebrate the months before your baby is born, remember, motherhood will bring its own sweet reward. Take time to honor and care for the wonderful woman you are right now!

9

LABOR *and* DELIVERY

Trust Your Body

Every time I read a pregnancy book or magazine article describing labor as an athletic event, I panicked. Did I really need the endurance of a triathlete to push my baby out? If this was true then I was in big trouble. Sure, I took a walk every night, but the last "athletic event" I participated in was high school gym class.

When the big day arrived, I was alternately nervous, excited, petrified, and thrilled to finally be meeting my daughter. During early labor, nagging doubts about my body's ability to step up to this intense physical challenge clouded my thoughts. However, once we checked into the hospital, my state of mind completely changed. Instead of more worried, I became strangely relaxed. I think what did it was the sense that wow, we're not leaving this place until the baby is born.

Labor quickly progressed and wave after wave of intensifying contractions seemed to unleash a power I never knew my body possessed. I felt stronger than I ever had in my entire life. Thoughts like "this is what my body is meant to do" and "I was born for this purpose" played repeatedly in my mind.

When time came to push, I gave it all I could. My energy levels never faltered. After about twenty minutes of pushing, my daughter's head emerged. I paused in the pushing as the midwife quickly suctioned my daughter's nose and mouth. It was like holding back a tidal wave. After she gave me the go ahead, I pushed again and with what felt like a mighty rush of energy leaving my body, Mia was born. I had done it! Instead of weak and out of shape, I felt powerful and exhilarated. I now know a plus-size woman's body can pulsate with vitality and strength. My daughter's birth was a double gift—a beautiful healthy newborn and a hefty dose of self-affirmation.

—SARAH, 32

TRUST IN YOUR body's ability to give birth. Whether your pregnancy has been smooth sailing or has encountered complications, don't doubt your own strength and perseverance. Approach labor and delivery with relaxed confidence knowing you have done everything within your control to make your pregnancy the healthiest it can be. If you are like the majority of all plus-size women, your childbirth experience will be completely normal *and* completely successful. Allow yourself to feel powerful. The birth of a child is one of life's most intense and rewarding experiences. Get excited! Your baby is almost here!

This chapter offers an overview of what plus-size women can expect during labor and delivery. You will find helpful information about pain relief/coping strategies and why your positive state of mind is so important for your childbirth experience. From worries about whether or not those skimpy hospital gowns will actually fit (or if they're even necessary) to unraveling the statistics behind elevated cesarean section rates among plus-size women, we answer your most pressing weight-related labor and delivery concerns.

Signs of Impending Labor

The night before I went into labor my body felt different, as though I had suddenly become lighter. I stayed up late that night, scurrying around the house cleaning and packing my bags for the hospital. After finally sleeping for a few hours, I woke to find my water had broken. A few hours later, the contractions started. It was all such a gradual, natural progression. My body knew just what to do.

—JESSICA, age 22

UNLESS YOU ARE having a scheduled induction, it's almost impossible to pinpoint just when labor will actually begin. Statistically, plus-size women are more likely to go past their due dates. For *all* women, due dates are only an approximation. Just 5 percent of babies are actually born on their predicted birthdays! How will you know the big moment has finally arrived—or is at least close at hand? Monitor your body for the following physical symptoms:

- **Lightening:** If breathing comes a little bit easier to you during the last few days of your pregnancy, heartburn diminishes, and you feel like your baby has dropped lower in your belly, you have most likely experienced lightening. Lightening occurs when your baby's head settles deep in your pelvis in preparation for birth. With your baby in this position, pressure you may have felt on your rib cage and upper intestinal tract is thankfully reduced. Lightening in first time mothers may occur a few weeks before birth. For experienced mothers, lightening may not occur until after labor has begun.

- **Loss of Mucous Plug:** Thick mucus protectively sealed your cervix for the past nine months. As your cervix *effaces* (thins and shortens) and *dilates* (opens), this mucous cap slides into the vagina, where you may eventually notice it as a clear or an opaque, pink, or slightly bloody vaginal discharge. Loss of the mucous plug is usually a good sign labor will soon begin, but is not always an accurate indicator. Some women may lose their mucous plugs weeks before giving birth. Others don't experience what is known as *show* (or "bloody show" if the mucus is tinged with blood) until labor contractions actually begin. Still, losing your mucous plug let's you know your body is making preparations for your baby's delivery.

- **Rupture of the amniotic sac:** Whether it's a gush of fluid or a constant trickle from your vagina, rupture of the amniotic sac is a sign labor is on its way. Check with your provider about what to do once your "water breaks" (call the office, report to hospital, etc.). Due to increased risk for infection, it is advised to refrain from doing things like taking a bath or having sex once the amniotic sac ruptures.

- **Contractions:** Increasingly strong and rhythmic uterine contractions are probably the most reliable—and hard to miss—sign that labor has truly begun. For reasons not completely known, your body signals for the release of *oxytocin*, a hormone responsible for stimulating your uterus to contract. When you first notice labor contractions, they may be as far apart as 15 to 20 minutes, last for 60 to 90 seconds, and feel like achy menstrual cramps.

Contractions gradually intensify and grow closer together as your uterine muscle works harder and harder to dilate your cervix. The regular squeezing of your uterus pushes your baby deeper into your pelvis. Pressure from your baby's head helps your cervix dilate.

The Three Stages of Labor

What was I thinking? Even after the first rumblings of labor contractions had started, I was so intent on seeing this one movie that I practically forced my best friend to see it with me. I convinced her that because labor took so long to progress in first-time mothers—and according to my childbirth educator, even longer in plus-size women—it would probably be the next day before any real action began. Was I ever wrong. Just after the previews ended I thought I would give birth right in the aisle. I called my doctor and my friend and I went straight to the hospital. By the time we got there I was seven centimeters dilated and in transition.

—VENICE, age 28

Labor is divided into three distinct stages. The first stage of labor lasts from the time your contractions start until your cervix is fully dilated to 10 cm (centimeters). Labor's second stage, also called the "pushing stage," doesn't end until your baby is born. During the third stage of labor, the placenta is expelled.

First Stage: Dilation

The first stage of labor is further broken down into three smaller phases: early labor, active labor, and transition:

EARLY LABOR PHASE
(CERVIX DILATES UP TO 4 CM IN DIAMETER)
- **Contractions:** Start approximately 15 to 20 minutes apart (or longer) and last 30 to 90 seconds each. By the end of early labor, contractions are about 5 minutes apart and last 45 to 60 seconds. Contractions may initially feel like menstrual cramps that keep getting stronger. You will probably be at home during this phase. Call your provider to report symptoms and gauge when you need to go to the hospital (or follow the plan you and your provider prearranged).

- **Changes in your body:** You may experience backache, diarrhea, leaking amniotic fluid (if the amniotic membrane has already ruptured), indigestion, a sensation of warmth in the abdomen, and/or "bloody show" (as your mucous plug now completely falls out it will probably be tinged with blood from broken capillaries in your cervix).
- **How you are feeling:** You will feel a mix of emotions, everything from exhilaration, joy, exuberance, to fear, anxiety, and worry.

ACTIVE LABOR PHASE
(CERVIX DILATES FROM 4 CM TO 7 CM IN DIAMETER)

- **Contractions:** Active labor contractions are more intense than those experienced at the end of early labor. Contractions last from 40 to 60 seconds and occur every 2 to 4 minutes.
- **Changes in your body:** You will find it more difficult to talk or walk during a contraction. You will probably experience back pain, achy legs, fatigue, and/or increased bloody show. You may also break out in a fine perspiration.
- **How you are feeling:** You may feel excited or relieved to finally be at the hospital or birthing center—there's no going back now! You may feel anxious about the growing intensity of labor contractions or completely focused on getting through each one.

TRANSITION PHASE (CERVIX DILATES FROM 7 CM UNTIL IT REACHES 10 CM IN DIAMETER)

- **Contractions:** As you achieve full dilation (10 cm), these are probably the most intense contractions you will experience. Fortunately, transition is usually the shortest phase of labor, lasting anywhere from 15 minutes to an hour or more. Contractions last between 60 to 90 seconds and are approximately 2 to 3 minutes apart.
- **Changes in your body:** You may experience hot flashes, leg cramps, shakes and chills, nausea or vomiting, bloody show, and increasing pressure in your lower back, rectum, and *perineum* (the skin between your vagina and anus).
- **How you are feeling:** You may be irritable or disoriented and not want to be touched or talked to during this very intense phase of labor. Some women may feel restless or frustrated if they feel the urge to bear down but can't because full dilation has not yet been reached.

Second Stage: Delivery

- **Contractions:** Contractions last from 60 to 90 seconds and are 2 to 5 minutes apart with a defined rest period in between. Now in the "pushing stage," you will bear down with each contraction.
- **Changes in your body:** An intense urge to push is triggered as your baby's head presses against your rectum and stretches out your vaginal and pelvic floor muscles. You may grunt as you bear down and will notice a burning sensation as your baby's head *crowns* (emerges).
- **How you are feeling:** Your emotions during this stage are usually linked with how well your pushing efforts are working. However, thanks to your body's release of endorphins (part of your body's pain relief system), when your baby is finally born, you will most likely feel euphoric!

Third Stage: Delivery of the Placenta

- **Contractions:** Contractions are mild and usually last less than a minute (they are minor compared to what you have experienced for the past few hours).
- **Changes in your body:** After your baby is born, the placenta detaches itself from the uterine wall and is delivered. Contractions then continue for a few minutes to help your uterus return to its prepregnancy size. You may still experience shakes. Vaginal bleeding will be heavy and clotted.
- **How you are feeling:** Still euphoric. By now you have probably held your baby and even nursed. Welcome to motherhood!

Plus-Size Concerns and Coping Strategies

PLUS-SIZE WOMEN, like women of all sizes, benefit from a prepared approach to childbirth. There are several ways you can gradually get ready for labor and delivery:

- **Discuss labor and delivery with your prenatal care provider.** Maintain an ongoing dialogue with your prenatal care provider about the health of your pregnancy. Your provider monitors your blood pressure, your weight gain, and your baby's growth and fetal heart rate. Ask your provider how this information will likely impact labor and delivery. Are you staying within the recommended weight-gain guidelines? Do you have a complication, such as gestational diabetes or preeclampsia, that may increase your chances for labor induction and/or cesarean delivery? If you had a cesarean section to deliver your first baby, is *vaginal birth after cesarean (VBAC)* an option for your current pregnancy? As your due date draws near your provider can interpret this information to give you a reasonable—but not always 100 percent accurate—idea about what to expect during your childbirth experience.

- **Keep taking good care of yourself.** Good prenatal nutrition remains important right up until the very end of your pregnancy. Avoid the common trap of grabbing too many fast-food meals as you rush around taking care of all the last-minute details before your baby arrives, or not eating enough out of nervousness about your approaching due date. Nutritious meals and snacks in the days leading up to the big event maintains your gradual weight gain and helps ensure you will make it through labor and delivery with energy to spare.

- **Attend childbirth education classes.** Learning about the birth process itself can ease your fears and help you feel more in control when labor actually begins. Childbirth education classes are usually offered through hospitals, community groups, birthing centers, or private individuals certified in a particular birthing method (such as Lamaze or the Bradley Method). Some women and their partners start taking classes almost as soon as they find out they're pregnant. You might decide holding off until the late second/early third trimester makes the information you will learn more relevant. However, don't wait until the third trimester to sign up for classes. Begin investigating education opportunities now and register before the course you want is full.

Depending on the topics covered, you might learn relaxation techniques, how your partner or loved one can best support you during labor, what to expect from a typical vaginal delivery, water birth, or cesarean delivery. Childbirth educators can answer your questions or refer you to other sources. If offered through a local hospital, you will go on a tour of the birthing wing and become acquainted with the amenities offered by the facility. Also, many women report childbirth education classes are an excellent opportunity to link up with other plus-size moms-to-be.

If you have time, maximize the number of classes you take and don't be afraid to attend those covering topics you consider uncomfortable. As one sister wisely put it, "I never entertained the notion that I wouldn't have the birth I wanted. When I ended up needing a cesarean section, the intense fear I experienced was definitely fear of the unknown. I recommend for women to be aware of all their options long before delivery. If your hospital or practice offers a free, one-night seminar on c-sections—just go. You will probably have a completely normal delivery but that little bit of knowledge goes a long way in keeping you calm and focused no matter what happens."

- **Consider doula support.** *Doulas* are professional labor assistants trained to provide hands-on assistance to women during childbirth. A doula is not a replacement for your partner's vital support, but is an additional source for continuous comfort. Depending on your needs, a doula may provide massage, recommend natural pain relief techniques, suggest alternative birthing positions, hold a hot or cold compress in place, or be there just to listen.

  Doulas have earned an excellent reputation in the past decade. Plus-size women, take note! According to medical research, women who are accompanied by a doula during childbirth actually have shorter labors, lower rates of cesarean sections, fewer forceps deliveries, and fewer episiotomies.

  In addition, studies show women who have doulas with them during labor are less likely to request medicated pain relief, such as an *epidural,* and are more likely to express satisfaction with their birthing experiences (so the doula's natural pain relief suggestions must really work!). Enlisting a doula's support might be just what you need to achieve the birthing experience you want.

  Three organizations certify most labor assistants: the Association of Labor Assistants and Childbirth Educators (ALACE), Doulas of North America (DONA), and the International Childbirth Educators Association (ICEA). These organizations are easily found on the Web and contain state-by-state directories. You can also call your hospital's maternity ward and ask if they can recommend any doulas in your area.

Some doulas work on a volunteer basis, but most charge anywhere from $200–400 for their labor and delivery services. See Resources for how to contact the above-listed organizations.

■ **Make a birth plan.** Many women write out a birth plan, a list of do's and don'ts tailored to fit their beliefs about normal childbirth. A birth plan might list the people you want present with you in the delivery room; state your desire to walk, shower, or take a bath during labor; indicate your stand on epidurals and other pain relief medications; and affirm your preference for delivery positions, such as squatting, lying on one side, sitting on a birthing stool, or having a water birth. Even a woman having a scheduled cesarean section can make a birth plan, writing out instructions for such things as lowering the surgical drape so she can see her baby being born.

Women report that creating these personalized statements about the moments surrounding their baby's birth helps them feel more actively involved and in control once they get to the delivery room. If you choose to write a birth plan, double-check with your prenatal care provider to make sure your wishes can be practically carried out (for example, candles cannot be lit in the hospital, as oxygen may be in use).

Your birthing experience is unique so stay realistic about following your plan once labor begins. Delivering your baby might be exactly what you visualized—or quite different. Make sure your birth plan is flexible enough to accommodate whatever situation might arise.

■ **Think positively and visualize a successful birth.** Feeling confidently relaxed about your body's ability to give birth can decrease your stress levels, reduce pain, and help you better focus on the hard work of labor and delivery. Women who actively practice relaxation and positive visualization techniques during childbirth typically report greater overall satisfaction with their birthing experiences. Women who are relaxed are less likely to experience fear and anxiety—negative feelings that can actually slow labor down. Even during a difficult labor, women who are less stressed out may be more willing to dig deep for that extra burst of energy needed to push the baby out.

The key to using relaxation techniques during labor is to start practicing them long before your due date arrives. Sit still in your favorite chair and focus on your breathing. Feel each breath enter and then leave your body. Start imagining each breath you take brings in something good (peace, love, energy) and each breath you let out releases a negative feeling from your body (stress, anxiety, fear). During labor you can change these thoughts to match your experience. Each breath in could be a mighty force guiding your baby further down into the birth canal; each breath out, the release of labor pain.

Some hospitals and independent childbirth educators offer classes in *hypnobirthing*, self-hypnosis techniques that work to reduce pain and fear by focusing the mind on staying calm and relaxed during labor. If you are panicked just thinking about your due date, this is probably a class worth taking.

How to Dress for Delivery

CHECKING INTO THE hospital just as labor contractions pick up steam—and just when you need to feel your most comfortable and confident—you are told to take off your clothes and put on a hospital gown. Problem? Standard-issue hospital gowns ("johnnies") are often too small for many plus-size women. If you want to walk the halls during labor, these gowns don't leave much to the imagination. Where's Lane Bryant when you really need her?

It might seem like a trivial issue, but small things like being given a hospital gown that obviously doesn't fit and then feeling obligated to wear it really does matter to your overall birthing experience. Hospital staff usually give women two gowns—one to cover the front and the other to cover the back. For plus-size women, wearing two too-small gowns is sometimes described as feeling very restrictive through the shoulders and arms.

Some sisters have called the labor and delivery unit and directly asked, do gowns come in larger sizes? Most of the time hospitals *do* have larger gowns available, so be sure to ask for one upon arrival. One no-nonsense sister went online and bought her own! As this plus-size woman reported, "it was the same ugly green color as the hospital one. When I was admitted and given their too-small johnny to wear, I simply slipped on my own. If anyone noticed, they never said anything."

Whether or not it's a perfect fit, is it even necessary for a laboring woman of any size to wear hospital-issue clothing? Unless hospital policies or medical reasons make putting on a hospital gown absolutely necessary (the advantage of a "johnny" is that it is easily removed in an emergency), you will probably be just fine wearing a loose, comfortable shirt brought from home, and your own bathrobe should you choose to walk the halls. Midwife training materials actually instruct midwives to encourage women to wear their own clothes during childbirth, even when they are laboring in a hospital. On the other hand, any clothing you wear during labor and delivery may become heavily soiled.

By the time labor gets intense, don't be surprised if you are like many women and prefer to wear nothing at all. In the meantime, don't forget to add "comfy labor clothes" to your must-pack list for the hospital.

Does Being Plus-Size Result in a Longer Labor?

MEDICAL RESEARCH SHOWS that—in general—plus-size women may spend a little more time in labor than the rest of the pregnant population. In one study of first time mothers, the dilation rate (how many centimeters the cervix opens per hour) was slightly slower than average in both overweight and obese women. Once contractions became regular, normal-BMI women took just over 6 hours to reach full dilation. In contrast, overweight women needed approximately 7 hours, and obese women took just under 8 hours to achieve the same results (when looked at individually, of course, plus-size experiences vary widely). Researchers noted the slow down most likely occurred during the early labor and active labor phases. During transition, women of all sizes dilated from 7 cm to 10 cm at approximately the same rate.

Though there are many theories, researchers still are not sure what exactly causes these lengthier first-stage labors. For whatever reason, it appears some plus-size women may simply require more contractions to fully dilate the cervix and best position their babies for delivery.

Your labor will hopefully be short and sweet, but spending a little longer than average in the first stage of labor probably doesn't indicate anything is wrong with your baby or your ability for a successful birth. If you have had no serious complications during your pregnancy and fetal heart monitoring shows your baby is tolerating labor well, your labor will most likely be left to progress at its own pace.

When Labor Is Too Slow

WHEN DILATION IS irregular or *much* slower than normal, your baby is not descending as expected, or if contractions just don't seem to be picking up steam, your provider will probably decide additional steps are needed to help your labor along. Some of these methods include:

- **Walk.** Unless for health/safety reasons you are confined to bed, walking during labor may make contractions more efficient. While medical studies vary on this topic, some experts believe walking slightly shifts the shape of your pelvis, making it wide enough to favor your baby's descent through the birth canal. Walking works with the force of gravity. More direct downward pressure from your baby's head helps push your cervix open wider during contractions.

  Compared with reclining in bed, walking also improves your circulation. Enhanced blood flow to your uterus means there is more fuel available to power your contractions (better blood flow also brings more oxygen and nutrients to your baby). Your partner can walk the halls of the maternity ward with you or assist you in climbing a flight of stairs.

- **Change positions.** Many women (and providers) swear by other gravity-friendly positions to move labor along, including slow dancing while leaning against your partner, standing up and leaning against a sturdy piece of furniture, or sitting on a birthing ball or birthing stool. Childbirth education classes usually offer many suggestions for effective laboring positions. Sometimes the childbirth educator will demonstrate or even practice techniques with you, so you will be more comfortable using them once the big day arrives.

- **Stay hydrated.** Dehydration slows down effective uterine contractions. Drink plenty of fluids during early and active labor to keep your contractions strong and regular (follow your provider's instructions about food and beverage choices). While staying hydrated is important, urinate frequently to keep your bladder as empty as possible. A full bladder may actually get in the way of your baby's descent!

- **Stay relaxed.** In some slow-moving labors, stress may be the underlying culprit. A woman of any size who enters childbirth fearful and anxious may trigger her body's "fight or flight response." When high levels of stress hormones (such as adrenaline) are released into the blood stream during early and active labor, blood flow is directed toward parts of the body that would be important should you need to flee. Blood flow is shifted to the skeletal muscles, those in the arms and legs, and away from where it is really needed—the uterus. Uterine muscle contractions might not get the power needed to operate at maximum capacity. Contractions slow down or become weaker as a result.

Women are often able to "turn off" their stress hormones and speed up their labors by practicing a variety of simple relaxation techniques. Take advantage of an early labor spent at home by doing the things you most enjoy. Bake some banana bread, watch your favorite movie, call your best friend, scrapbook, write in your journal, or go for a walk.

Once you check in at the hospital or birthing center, have your partner give you a massage and listen to soothing music together. If you get the go-ahead from your provider, take a warm bath or shower. Use your focused breathing techniques. Meditate or pray. Practice positive visualization—with each contraction visualize your cervix opening up like a flower in the morning sun.

Medical Intervention

If labor is still off track, despite your best efforts, medical methods are available to speed labor up (aka *augment* labor). When the cervix dilates less then 1 cm per hour during active labor, your provider may decide to rupture your amniotic sac, if it is still intact. What looks like a long plastic crochet hook will be used to break the bag of waters. You will probably feel the same kind of pressure associated with a pelvic exam. Studies show labor can be reduced an average of 2 hours after the amniotic sac is ruptured.

Another common method to augment labor is to start an intravenous drip of *pitocin,* the synthetic form of oxytocin (a hormone your body produces during labor). Pitocin works quickly to make contractions stronger. Cervical dilation should increase as a result. Pitocin is a powerful drug. Your baby's heartbeat will most likely be monitored continuously once a "pit drip" is started.

Medical intervention during labor is controversial. Current statistics show that more than 50 percent of all women have their labors somehow medically sped up. Many women are left to wonder if their slower labors are not given the chance to naturally progress and if medical intervention is turned to too quickly—especially when no other signs point to anything being wrong. Discuss labor augmentation with your provider long before your due date. Get a sense of what signs your provider looks for to assess your labor's effectiveness. If you have a complication such as preeclampsia or gestational diabetes, talk to your provider about how these conditions might change expectations.

Coping with Labor Pain

LABOR PAIN IS different. It's pain with a purpose. If you have ever climbed a mountain and dragged yourself up those last few steps to the summit because you knew you would get the view of a lifetime, what you experienced is a lot like labor. Every contraction, however intense, is bringing you one step closer to your baby. You may be able to sleep through early labor or distract yourself from mild pain by watching a movie or going for a walk. As contractions grow more intense, however, use more specific pain-relief strategies. There are many effective, easy to use, and all-natural pain relief techniques to reduce discomfort during labor. Many women report trying a potpourri of techniques, whereas others just stick with the first one that really worked well. These include:

- **Heat:** When you pack for the hospital, include a heating pad and hot water bottle. Reduce labor pain by applying heat to your lower back, shoulders, thighs, perineum, or lower abdomen. Heat helps alleviate pain because it increases blood flow and relaxes muscles. One rule of thumb, heating devices should feel hot but never burn. Don't apply anything to your body that is too uncomfortably hot to hold in your hands.
- **Cold:** Some like it hot and others like it cold when it comes to pain relief. Cold numbs pain because it slows down neurotransmitters from telling your brain that you hurt. If you experience back pain during labor, have your partner apply a cold pack to your lower back to see if this offers some relief. Don't have a cold pack? Frozen wet wash cloths, a freezer bag filled with ice, or a frozen 16-ounce plastic bottle of water can be placed on virtually any body part that needs relief.
- **Counterpressure:** If you took a childbirth education class on pain relief, you learned about counterpressure when the instructor took out the tennis balls and rolling pins and had your partner practice with them to give you a back massage. Counterpressure works by massaging or pressing against the area where pain is felt. Instead of focusing on the pain, your

brain concentrates on this new sensation. During real labor, the light massage you and your partner probably giggled through in class won't seem so silly. It won't be so light, either. Aggressive pressure is sometimes needed to achieve relief and may even cause a few black and blue marks.

- **Relaxation techniques:** The same bag of tricks you use to stay calm during labor also work to relieve pain. Focused breathing, positive visualization, meditation, prayer . . . any of these can give you somewhere else to mentally concentrate when labor pains strike. Hypnobirthing is a form of self-hypnosis that helps women avoid pain by entering a trance-like state of deep relaxation during labor. Check for hypnobirthing training classes in your area.

- **Hydrotherapy:** Taking a warm shower or a bath can target a certain area or bring all-over muscle relaxation. Sitting backward on a folding chair placed in the shower and simply letting the water stream down on the lower back often provides welcome relief. Some women want to take a shower or bath, but don't think this is possible because they are hooked up to a fetal monitor. Depending on how well labor progresses, your provider might switch to intermittent monitoring—checking fetal heart rate and contraction strength every 15 minutes or so. This gives you a chance to take a quick shower or bath. Even a few minutes of hydrotherapy can ease discomfort.

Induction

Induced labor, when uterine contractions are jump-started through medication or other means, is often chosen when an immediate or planned delivery is in the best interest of both mother and child. Because plus-size women have higher than average rates of preeclampsia and gestational diabetes, two complications sometimes requiring the delivery of the baby before the due date, plus-size women also have higher-than-average rates of induced labors.

Labor is most often induced in the hospital under the supervision of your provider (or attending OB) and may include the following steps:

- **Ripening the cervix:** The cervix must be soft ("ripe") before it can efface and dilate. To ripen the cervix, *prostaglandin* gel is applied or a prostaglandin tablet is placed in the vagina.

Prostaglandin is a hormone responsible for preparing the cervix for labor. Your cervix is checked a few hours after the prostaglandin is applied. If effacement and dilation have not started, more prostaglandin may be applied. For some women, prostaglandin is powerful enough on its own to get labor started.

- **Administering pitocin:** Once the cervix is ripe and has begun to dilate, an IV drip of pitocin is started. As pitocin circulates through your bloodstream, it stimulates the uterine muscle to contract. You will wear an electronic fetal monitor on your belly to measure contraction strength and your baby's heart rate. A nurse or doctor must be continuously available to supervise how you and your baby respond to the pitocin. The level of pitocin in the IV drip can be raised or lowered depending on how your contractions progress.
- **Rupturing the amniotic sac:** If the bag of waters has not already broken, your provider will do the job at some point during your labor (before or after the pitocin drip is started). Rupturing the amniotic membrane helps labor progress. Like prostaglandin gel, this is sometimes the only induction method needed to get contractions underway.

Induced labors are generally shorter than average labors for both first-time and experienced mothers. Women who have labor induced often feel overwhelmed by how quickly contractions progress. Practice relaxation and other natural pain-relief techniques to deal with anxiety and physical discomfort. Request medicated pain relief if you choose. Enlist your partner to provide massage and moral support.

When labor is induced, your baby's heart rate is closely monitored. Some hospitals offer more advanced monitoring equipment that allow for greater freedom of movement, but most rely on traditional double-belt external fetal monitors. Especially if you have been in bed for a while, you may start feeling a little stir crazy. If your labor is progressing smoothly and your baby shows no heart rate irregularities, you can probably negotiate some time away from the monitor to take a walk or shower.

If your baby shows signs of heart rate irregularities or if your health shows signs of deterioration—for example, your blood pressure spikes if you have preeclampsia—your provider may decide a cesarean section is the best option. The majority of women who have their labors induced, however, go on to have completely normal vaginal deliveries.

One sister reflected on her induction experience as follows, "I was induced because I had gestational diabetes, was almost a week past my due date, and an ultrasound showed my amniotic fluid levels had dropped too low. Having my labor induced was like watching one of those videos from childbirth class on fast forward. Everything was quick, even the delivery. I was in hard labor for about five hours and then pushed for about fifteen minutes before my son was born. He was totally healthy and had no problems with his blood sugar."

FETAL MONITORING: HOW'S YOUR BABY DOING?

YOUR BLOOD PRESSURE and other vital signs are monitored throughout labor. The only way to adequately evaluate how well your baby tolerates labor is to monitor your baby's heart rate and his or her response to contractions. You will notice that your baby's heart rate varies quite a bit over time. Most of these variations are completely normal and not cause for concern. Options for fetal monitoring include:

- **Auscultation:** *Auscultation* means listening to your baby's heartbeat at intermittent intervals (every hour, every 20 minutes, etc.). Timing of auscultation is dictated by the stage of labor and any risk factors. Your provider or a nurse may use either a handheld Doppler ultrasound device or a special type of stethoscope called a *fetoscope* to evaluate your baby's heart rate. Your baby's heartbeat will be listened to before, during, and after a contraction.
- **Continuous external fetal monitoring:** This type of monitoring provides an ongoing record of how your baby responds to labor and is frequently used in induced labors and high risk deliveries. Belts are strapped around your belly to hold two monitoring devices in place. One measures your baby's heartbeat, the other records timing and intensity of contractions. Results are printed out on a tracing strip.
- **Internal monitoring:** This method of fetal monitoring only works once your amniotic sac has ruptured. To obtain your baby's heart rate, an electrode (long, flexible wire) is inserted into your vagina and placed against your baby's scalp. An intrauterine catheter is also inserted to measure contraction strength. The advantage of internal monitoring is its ability to provide precise measurements.

continued

> ● **Telemetry:** With *telemetry*, a type of continuous monitoring, a small device placed on your thigh uses radio waves to transmit your baby's heartbeat to a receiver at the nurses' station. The main benefit of telemetry is that it allows you to maintain full mobility during labor. Ask your provider about whether or not telemetry is an option where you will deliver.

Epidurals

EPIDURAL ANESTHESIA NUMBS the lower half of your body and prevents you from feeling most of the pain from labor contractions. Stronger epidurals are frequently used in cesarean deliveries. When an epidural is administered, you sit or lie on your side and curve your back outward. An anesthesiologist inserts a needle into your lower back between two of the lumbar vertebrae. After the needle is placed close to the spinal canal (called the epidural space), a catheter is inserted through the needle. The needle is removed, but the catheter remains in the epidural space. An anesthetic is continuously administered for the remainder of labor and delivery. The catheter is removed shortly after birth.

Anxiety about failed epidural placement is common among plus-size women. Fortunately, the medical community understands this concern. To make sure anesthesia is accurately and efficiently administered, the American College of Obstetricians and Gynecologists now recommends for plus-size women to meet with an anesthesiologist just after admission to the hospital during labor (or during a late–third trimester prenatal appointment). This consultation gives the anesthesiologist an opportunity to evaluate your body type and determine whether special techniques are needed if you request an epidural or require one for cesarean delivery. In the rare case general anesthesia is administered during a cesarean delivery, the anesthesiologist can check ahead of time to see if slightly different equipment should be used.

Meeting with an anesthesiologist is *not* meant to pressure you into choosing medicated pain relief during what is otherwise a completely normal labor. Plus-size women do not require pain relief in noncesarean deliveries unless it is their preference.

What Is Abdominal Lifting?

IN PLUS-SIZE women with very relaxed abdominal walls (sometimes called a "pendulous abdomen"), there is a chance the baby will be slightly out of line with the pelvic opening. Even a small misalignment could cause a slow down in labor because the baby is less able to properly descend. A simple technique called *abdominal lifting* is sometimes employed by plus-size women during a slower first-stage labor to help better position their babies.

In this maneuver, you stand upright and lace your fingers just below your belly. Slightly bend your knees and tilt your pelvis forward. It helps to lean against a wall or be supported by your partner while doing this. As a contraction starts, lift your belly upward (about 1 to 2 inches) and then inward (about an inch). Hold this lift through the contraction, lowering your belly as the contraction fades. When successful, this technique helps your baby to put more pressure on the cervix. One disadvantage to abdominal lifting is that it is often tiring for a laboring woman to maintain this position.

The abdominal lift is used during a slow-to-progress labor and not one already moving along at a fast clip. If you see a midwife for care or have hired a doula to be with you during labor, they will most likely be very knowledgeable about abdominal lifting and can make sure you use the correct technique. Some doulas tie a scarf around the mother's neck and belly as a makeshift sling to hold the belly up and leave the hands free. Many OBs are also familiar with these alternative positions for helping labor along. Discuss with your provider whether or not abdominal lifting is right for you.

WHERE IS YOUR BABY DURING LABOR?

WITH EACH UTERINE contraction, your baby is pushed deeper and deeper into your pelvis. Keeping track of where your baby's head is in relation to bony landmarks on either side of the pelvis (these are called the *ischial spines*) gives a pretty good idea of how well contractions are moving your baby along. Locating your baby's position can be done through digital vaginal exam. Progress through your pelvic outlet is measured in stations:

−3 Station: Baby's head is just entering the pelvis.

0 Station: Baby's head has dropped into the pelvis.

+3 Station: Baby's head is near the opening of your vagina.

The Power of Pushing

WHEN YOU FEEL the intense urge to push, you will probably be stunned by the power your body exhibits. Researchers have found that to deliver their babies, plus-size women need to push an average of 15 minutes *less* than do thinner women! Good proof to dispel the myth you need nothing short of abs of steel in order to give birth.

Pushing creates intraabdominal pressure that works with uterine contractions to propel your baby closer and closer to birth. And yes, it does feel very similar to straining during a bowel movement. Some babies are born after two pushes and some are born after two or more hours of bearing down during contractions. For women of all sizes, and especially for first-time mothers, it is almost impossible to gauge ahead of time exactly how long delivery will take.

Chances are excellent you will have a successful delivery and your baby will be here before you know it. Helpful ways to maximize your pushing efforts include:

- **Push with the urge.** After you have reached complete dilation (10 cm) and the powerful need to push kicks in, take a deep breath and bear down with your next contraction. Some women bear down during the entire contraction, and others may push a few times. Release as the contraction begins to fade. Bearing down when you are not having a contraction does very little to move your baby along and can more quickly tire you out. If you need to grunt or moan, follow your instincts and don't hold back. Your body is performing intense work and you may need to let off a little steam.
- **Get into position.** A hot topic in most childbirth classes is whether the standard hospital position for giving birth—body slightly elevated while lying in bed, legs spread and lifted, feet braced against supports—is the best position. Alternatives such as squatting, sitting on a birthing stool, or sitting upright in bed, enlist the aid of gravity to help you while you push. Although research is divided on whether it is better to give birth in these gravity-friendly positions, women themselves report that birthing in an upright position decreases pain. Plus-size women with gestational hypertension or preeclampsia may benefit from a left-side lying position to lower blood pressure during delivery. In this position, your partner lifts and holds your right leg as you push.

Experiment with different birthing positions during delivery. This is especially recommended if progress is slow—one advantage to *not* having an epidural is the ability to move around or stand up during childbirth. Whatever position you choose, make sure it is one in which you feel comfortable.

- **Rest between contractions.** As much as you are able, consciously relax between each contraction. Breathe in and out slowly several times during these rest periods to stay calm and oxygenate your blood. Your baby still relies on your bloodstream for oxygen even in these last few moments before birth.

- **Feel encouraged.** This is a great chance for your partner's inner cheerleader to emerge. Pushing is hard work and hearing some reassuring words lets you know your efforts are working. After an hour of pushing you can get a much-needed second wind when you hear your partner call out, "I see the baby's head!"

  Keep your own thoughts positive. Repeating a simple key phrase when bearing down, such as "My body is strong" or "I'm open," may decrease your body's stress response and give you a little more pushing power.

- **Avoid tearing.** As your baby's head pushes closer to birth, your perineum begins to bulge. Pressure from your baby's head as it crowns may tear the perineum in one or more locations. Since plus-size women tend to have larger babies, tearing might be something you are more likely to encounter. To help protect the perineum from tears, many midwives and doulas provide perineal massage during labor and delivery. Massage may loosen the perineum, allowing it to stretch and stay intact as your baby is born (some women practice perineal massage at home for a few weeks before their due dates).

  Another helpful technique is for your partner or doula to hold a hot compress to your perineum during delivery, enhancing the perineum's ability to relax and stretch. Applying heat also reduces the burning or stinging sensations felt in this area during birth.

  When the baby's head crowns and your urge to push is at its strongest, you may be asked to pause in your pushing to allow the perineum to stretch. You may also be asked to push when you do not have a contraction, in an effort to avoid a tear. Any tears are stitched up after your baby is born and the placenta delivered. Applying ice to the perineum after birth can provide relief from pain.

Your provider may decide to perform an episiotomy, widening the vaginal opening by making an incision into the perineum. This is done during delivery if there is reason to believe your baby needs to be delivered quickly. An anesthetic is applied to the perineum before an episiotomy is performed.

- **If you have had an epidural:** Depending on the amount of sensation you feel in the lower half of your body, you may or may not feel the powerful urge to push. Bearing down may be more of a voluntary effort on your part. Your provider will probably give you explicit instructions on when to start and stop pushing.

And then, no matter how long labor lasted or how many times you pushed, it's over. Your beautiful baby is born! Take time to revel in everything your body just accomplished.

A sister reflected on her own transformation during birth, "Before going into labor I worried that my negative feelings toward my body would stop me from really letting go and giving myself over to the birthing process. One of the most amazing parts of labor and delivery was completely forgetting about the fact that I'm fat. After years of carefully covering my body, it just felt better to strip off my clothes when things got intense. I didn't give it a second thought. I howled and moaned and even laughed uncontrollably after a particularly intense contraction. I pushed like there was no tomorrow.

"Who was this uninhibited woman? It certainly wasn't the quiet, shy person who thought anyone who looked at her must be thinking about what size she wears. My doctor stopped back in the room to check on me and the baby a few hours after delivery. He told me I came through childbirth 'like a rock star.' I love that description."

Plus-Size Women and Cesarean Deliveries

DELIVERY BY *cesarean section* is sometimes the safest choice for both you and your baby. According to current statistics, plus-size women give birth by cesarean section more often than normal weight women do.

Why the higher rates? Women who have their labors induced are at increased risk for cesarean delivery and plus-size women are more likely to require induction of labor for such problems as preeclampsia and gestational diabetes. Plus-size women generally deliver larger babies, especially if they gain more weight than recommended or develop gestational diabetes. Women who deliver high-birth-weight babies also have an increased chance to give birth via cesarean section.

When researchers grouped together plus-size women without any pregnancy complications, their cesarean section rates mirrored that of normal weight women. It appears that the higher frequency of cesarean sections among plus-size women who experience certain health problems during pregnancy raises the cesarean average for the general plus-size population.

(It is important to note: Plus-size women who are able to successfully manage their complications, such as by following a diet and exercise program if they have gestational diabetes, often drop their risk for cesarean delivery back to the "normal" rate.)

Women of all sizes, whether or not they ever develop complications during pregnancy, should become informed about cesarean delivery. Discuss with your OB well ahead of time what reasons would lead to the decision for a cesarean (problems described above, as well as a breech baby, multiple-birth pregnancy, placenta previa, hemorrhage, or a previous history of a cesarean section). If you go into labor and your provider determines a cesarean section is needed to deliver your baby, make sure you understand the reasons why. Some plus-size women worry that excess abdominal fat will make a cesarean section more difficult to perform. Discuss this fear with your provider to get a more realistic picture of what you could expect.

Your cesarean may have been planned weeks in advance, or take place after a long time spent in labor. No matter when the decision is made, the steps to delivering your baby are basically the same:

- **Prepping:** An IV drip is started prior to any anesthesia. Needed fluids and medications will be given through the IV. If one is not already there, you will have an epidural or spinal block put in place. The anesthesiologist will administer a stronger dose of anesthetic than you would normally receive during a vaginal delivery (general anesthesia has become increasingly rare). To keep your bladder empty, a catheter is inserted through your urethra into your bladder. The upper portion of your pubic hair may be shaved and your abdomen is washed with a disinfectant. A drape is placed just below your shoulders to maintain a sterile environment around the incision site.

- **Your partner:** Unless a serious emergency dictates otherwise, once you are prepped your partner can be at your side, dressed in surgical scrubs, ready to provide support.
- **Delivery:** When the cesarean is performed, the abdomen is entered in layers. Your doctor usually makes a horizontal incision just at or above the pubic hairline (in some plus-size women with heavy abdomens, a vertical or horizontal incision higher up on the abdomen may be used). Your abdominal muscles are spread apart—not cut. Another incision is made to enter the abdominal cavity and gain access to the uterus. A final incision is made in the uterus and your baby is lifted out. The umbilical cord is clamped and cut. The placenta is removed before the incisions are stitched closed.
- **Birth:** Some women request the drape be lowered for their baby's birth—or you can use a mirror to witness your baby's arrival. After birth, your partner or a nurse can bring your baby to you. Depending on how you feel physically, you can hold your baby (some "wonder women" report breastfeeding their newborns—with a little assistance—right on the operating table!). To decrease your risk for surgical infection, a dose of antibiotics is given just after delivery.
- **Recovery:** After a complication-free cesarean section you will return to your room for recovery (though not typical, in very obese women there is higher risk for longer operating times and increased blood loss). Varying strength pain medication is administered. Barring any health concerns, you will be able to "room in" with your baby. Take advantage of your slightly longer stay in the hospital (most likely 2 to 4 days) to receive breast-feeding support. Lactation consultants on staff can show you comfortable positions that don't place stress on your stitches.

What is it like emotionally when you have a c-section? As described by this sister, "I had preeclampsia from about the 20th week of pregnancy. Because my blood pressure kept creeping higher and my baby's growth was slowing down, my doctor decided at 35 weeks that a cesarean section was needed. I was nervous. I cried. And then I decided to just get over it. This was my baby's birth! The moment I had been dreaming about for all these many months. Before leaving for the hospital we grabbed our favorite CDs and a small boom box. We thought it'd be nice to unwind after the operation by listening to music. When my doctor found out we had brought the CDs, she insisted we play some music during the actual delivery. My daughter was born halfway through the Beatles' *Rubber Soul* album. So, my memory of having a cesarean? Feeling nothing from the waist down, listening to my doctor sing along to 'Norwegian Wood,' hearing my baby's first sweet cry, and then finally holding my daughter in my arms. Slightly changing the lyrics from another favorite song, if you can't have the birth you want, love the birth you get."

CONGRATULATIONS! Your baby has finally arrived! For more on newborn care, recovery issues, and how plus-size women can best bounce back after birth, see chapter 10, "Beautiful Beginnings."

10

BEAUTIFUL BEGINNINGS:
Postpartum Life

Momentum

My motivation to eat right and exercise during pregnancy was a healthy baby. Now my motivation is the future. I want to give my daughter the best possible start in life. I want to enjoy being a mother. Most of all, I want to show my daughter what it means to be a strong, healthy woman.

—KRISTEN, age 29

MAKING THE COMMITMENT to eat right and exercise, actively participating in your health care, loving and trusting your body . . . these are life-altering accomplishments. You have got a lot of momentum as you enter motherhood. Make the positive choices you have worked so hard to achieve over these last nine months become a permanent part of your new life.

This chapter features the postpartum issues most relevant to plus-size women: what to expect as you recover from childbirth, why breast-feeding is so important for you and your baby, how to begin a gradual postpartum weight-loss program, and how to recognize the warning signs of postpartum depression. You will also learn practical steps for raising a healthy, active child.

Over the past nine months, your plus-size pregnancy has reaffirmed your ability to take excellent care of yourself. You have put extraordinary effort into making your pregnancy a success. What follows is the next part of your journey: putting yourself, your baby, and your new family on the road to a happy, healthy life together.

Recovering from Birth

YOU ARE EXHAUSTED, exhilarated, ravenous . . . you have just given birth! When you hold your newborn for the first time, it's amazing to think that this fragile being is now yours to love and care for—forever! In the midst of counting and recounting those ten tiny fingers and toes, however, don't forget about your own body. You just went through nine months of pregnancy and several hours of labor. Your body needs time to recuperate from pregnancy and childbirth.

The first six weeks or so after birth is called the postpartum period. While every woman recovers from childbirth in her own way, you will most likely notice several physical changes as your body returns to its prepregnant state.

Here's what you can expect:

- **Weight loss:** One of the first changes you may notice after giving birth is how much lighter you feel. Most plus-size women experience a 10- to 15-pound weight loss immediately after birth—the combined weight of the baby, placenta, and amniotic fluid. As blood volume and other body fluids rapidly return to nonpregnant levels, a few more pounds of pregnancy weight are shed. Plus-size women who stayed within the recommended weight-gain guidelines during pregnancy often report weighing a little less a few weeks after giving birth than they did before becoming pregnant.
- **Uterine contractions:** As your uterus shrinks back to a nonpregnant size, you may experience mild to painful contractions for approximately the first week following birth. Called *afterpains,* contractions are usually more pronounced in women who have given birth before. To help with discomfort, apply a hot water bottle or heating pad to your abdominal area (don't let these heating objects come in contact with your baby). Your provider might suggest ibuprofen or acetaminophen for pain relief.
- **Vaginal bleeding:** As your uterus squeezes back to its normal size, the uterus's thickened lining is shed. Known as *lochia,* vaginal bleeding in the first few days postpartum resembles

heavy menstrual flow and is bright red. Lochia eventually becomes lighter, finally tapering off by about the fourth postpartum week. However, it is not unusual for lochia to continue for up to eight weeks or for bleeding to turn into a yellowish discharge. Contact your provider if you notice any of the following symptoms: vaginal bleeding that is light and then suddenly turns heavy and bright red again, or vaginal discharge that contains unusually large blood clots or smells foul.

PLUS-SIZE HINT: While you are in the hospital, you will probably be offered a pair of disposable mesh panties to wear after you give birth. These hold pads in place to absorb the heavy postbirth discharge and can be conveniently tossed after use. Many sisters report that these panties don't live up to their "one-size-fits-all" label. When deciding what belongings to take with you to the hospital, pack several pairs of panties you don't mind ruining or throwing away.

- **Soreness in the perineum:** The perineum stretched and possibly tore during delivery, or maybe you had an episiotomy. As a result, your perineum may feel swollen, bruised, and sore in the first few days after giving birth. Applying cold packs helps reduce swelling and pain. Your provider may give you a numbing cream/spray or recommend you use witch hazel pads to ease discomfort. These same techniques work for hemorrhoid pain.

  Another alternative is to take a *sitz bath*. Hydrotherapy is a natural, time-tested method to relieve aches and pains. Simply fill the tub with a few inches of warm water (enough to cover your hips) and soak your perineum. In the first few days after giving birth, have someone on hand in case you need help getting in and out of the tub. Pat your perineum dry with a clean cloth after you bathe.

  You can buy a portable sitz bath at most pharmacies (the hospital may give you one). It's a small plastic dish placed over the toilet and filled with water. Portable sitz baths hold just enough water to cover your perineum. Filling the sitz bath with cold rather than warm water may provide a greater level of pain relief.

  If you have stitches from an episiotomy or tear, wash with a squirt bottle instead of wiping after you urinate (ask the nurse for a device called a peri-bottle). Pat the area dry with toilet paper or a clean cloth. Wiping from front to back after a bowel movement protects a healing episiotomy or tear from becoming infected by bacteria from the rectum.

Performing Kegels is one of the easiest and fastest ways to help the perineum regain its former shape and tone. Because these exercises strengthen the pelvic floor, Kegels may prevent urinary incontinence, another common side effect of childbirth. See page 136 for basic instructions.

- **Increased urination:** As blood volume returns to prepregnancy levels, excess fluids are no longer needed. As a result, you will notice an increased need to urinate for approximately the first few days after delivery.

- **Constipation and gas pains:** Labor slows down the movement of food through the intestinal tract and often leads to postpartum bloating and constipation. Going a day or more without eating anything substantial, side effects from pain relief medications, and staying in bed for long periods of time are other common causes for bowel movement irregularities. Some women may be afraid to have bowel movements due to pain from an episiotomy or hemorrhoids.

  Relieve constipation and gas pressure by eating plenty of high-fiber foods as part of your postpartum diet (high-fiber fruits, vegetables, and whole grains are good choices). Moving around as soon as you can after birth helps to restart bowel movements. Drinking plenty of water keeps stools soft. Brew up some peppermint tea, a natural remedy for bloating and gas pain. Discomfort should pass within a few days.

- **Hormonal changes:** As estrogen levels drop after delivery, hormonal fluctuations may cause you to experience night sweats for several weeks after giving birth (night sweats are also common later in life during menopause). Keep your bedroom cool while you sleep, and place a towel underneath you to absorb any perspiration.

- **Breast engorgement:** Delivering the placenta provides your breasts with a hormonal wakeup call to begin breast milk production. When your milk "comes in," about two to four days after delivery, it's normal for breasts to feel very full, hard, and tender (called *engorgement*). Large-breasted women may only notice that their breasts feel heavier. The easiest relief for engorgement is to breastfeed your baby. As you establish a nursing relationship with your newborn, your milk supply regulates itself and engorgement diminishes.

If after careful consideration you choose not to nurse, apply ice packs to your breasts and wear a support bra or chest binder to relieve swelling and discomfort. In women who choose not to breastfeed, severe engorgement should not last longer than a few days. The many benefits of breastfeeding and how to start breastfeeding your baby are discussed a little further on in this chapter.

- **Exhaustion:** Many factors combine to make new mothers fatigued and worn out: a long and difficult labor, recovering from a cesarean section, the normal blood loss that accompanies childbirth, a newborn who confuses night and day. . . . While you probably can't avoid exhaustion altogether, some helpful steps to get some well-deserved rest include:

  - *Limit visitors while you are at the hospital.* It's nice to have company, but too many visitors interferes with your ability to rest. Because you are only at the hospital for about two days for a vaginal birth, or three to four days for a cesarean delivery, stick to a small guest list. Tell everyone else you will post lots of pictures on the Internet (put your partner in charge of spreading the word). Plan a date in the near future for family and friends to come see your new bundle of joy.
  - *Get help.* Enlist your partner, family member, or a close friend to help out with daily chores and cooking once you come home from the hospital. Your attention during the first few days and weeks postpartum should be focused on taking care of your baby and making sure you get enough rest. Let someone else worry about the dusting and vacuuming.
  - *Sleep when your baby sleeps.* Use naptime as a chance to catch up on your sleep and not the household chores. Move the bassinet or crib into your room so you will hear your baby when he or she wakes up. If you are a heavy sleeper, make sure someone else is around to wake you up in case your baby's cries are not enough of an alarm clock.
  - *Breastfeed.* Breast milk is ready anytime, anywhere. Once you come home from the hospital, breastfeeding eliminates energy-zapping trips to the store and extra time spent preparing formula and washing bottles. Another breastfeeding perk—being able to nurse your baby while lying down!

If you had an uncomplicated delivery, you probably won't see your provider again until your postpartum checkup (four to six weeks after giving birth). Expect a standard gynecological exam. Your provider makes sure stitches from an episiotomy or tear are dissolved, and that your uterus has returned to a nonpregnant size. If you had gestational diabetes, you will need one more screening test to make sure blood glucose levels are back within normal range.

Your provider also wants to know how you are adjusting to motherhood and answer any questions you may have about this major life transition. If you are physically and emotionally ready to start having sex again, discuss birth control options with your provider. For breastfeeding women, certain birth control options may be better choices than others (the mini-pill and Depo Provera are considered compatible with breastfeeding). If you have used a diaphragm in the past for birth control, you will need to be refitted now that you have given birth. For those women who used an IUD (intrauterine device) before trying to conceive, you can arrange for another to be put in place.

Recovering from a Cesarean Section

Besides the standard physical changes and discomforts that accompany giving birth, recovering from a cesarean section carries with it a special set of challenges and concerns. Because you have just had major abdominal surgery, you will most likely stay in the hospital for three or four days after your baby is born. This gives your provider the ability to examine the incision site numerous times and evaluate how well the healing process is beginning.

Some plus-size women may need the surgical sutures or clips left in place for a longer period of time to make sure the wound is fully closed (7 to 10 days rather than 4 days). Your provider will determine what best suits your needs. Most sutures dissolve on their own.

Other cesarean recovery issues include:

- **Urinary discomfort:** A catheter inserted through your urethra during surgery drained your bladder and kept it out of the way during your baby's delivery. Once the catheter is removed (usually twelve hours after surgery), you may experience irritation or pain when you attempt to urinate. Discomfort can be mild to moderate and may last up to a few days. Stay as relaxed as possible when you urinate and drink plenty of water.

  Catheterization also leads to increased risk for urinary tract infections. Report any of the following symptoms to your provider: itching or burning sensations, frequent urination of only small amounts of urine, feeling the need to urinate all the time, pain in your kidneys (felt as mid-back pain), or fever.

- **Surgical area:** Plus-size women who carried extra weight in the abdominal area prepregnancy are at greater risk for developing an infection at the incision site. A fold of skin overhanging the healing scar can create a moist, warm environment—the perfect breeding ground for bacteria. You must pay very close attention to keeping the incision clean and dry. While you are in the hospital, your provider (or one of the nurses) will give you specific instructions on how you to take care of your healing incision once you go home.

  If at any time you notice red, oozing, and/or shooting pain in the area around the incision, or you develop a fever, immediately notify your provider. One sister gave the following tip, "a hair dryer turned to the 'cool' setting works wonders to keep the scar dry."

- **Pain management:** Your incision site will feel very sore and tender for the first few days after delivery (pain should gradually lessen). While in the hospital, initial pain relief may come in the form of an intravenous narcotic. Once you are able to take food, you will receive oral pain medications. Most oral pain medications are compatible with breastfeeding.

- **Getting back on your feet:** When the epidural anesthetic has worn off, you will probably be able to stand up and—with assistance—slowly begin to move around. As much as you are able to, be mobile. Movement helps your intestines start working again and relieves gas pains (sometimes very intense after a cesarean). Simply walking slowly around your hospital room a few times improves your circulation and reduces the likelihood of blood clots forming in your legs (a problem associated with staying in bed for long periods of time). You will most likely be able to get out of bed within twelve to twenty-four hours of delivery.

- **Breastfeeding:** Women who give birth by cesarean section are capable of successfully breastfeeding their babies. Make sure your provider and the nurses on duty know you want to breastfeed. Begin rooming-in with your baby as soon as you can (the day after surgery or earlier depending on how you feel and hospital policy). This closeness makes breastfeeding more convenient for both of you. You may feel more comfortable if your partner or a close family member remains with you and your baby. Your support person can lift and change the baby and help you get into position for nursing.

Breastfeeding your baby early and often ensures a good milk supply. Ask one of the hospital's lactation consultants, often an RN who is specially trained in breastfeeding issues, to show you breastfeeding positions that don't place pressure on your stitches. The two most common positions—side-lying nursing and the football hold—are described later in this chapter.

- **Postpartum support:** Because you just had surgery, it's normal to feel wiped out. Arrange for someone to be on hand during the first few weeks to help you out around the house. Avoid heavy lifting or straining for approximately six weeks after giving birth. This lessens excess pressure on the incision and gives it a better chance to heal. Until your provider gives you the okay to resume these activities, let your partner heft the infant car seat and leave the laundry baskets in the basement for someone else to lug upstairs.

In addition to physical recovery, many women require emotional healing after a cesarean section. It's not uncommon for women who deliver their babies by cesarean section to feel cheated or let down by their childbirth experiences. After all the anticipation of labor and delivery, it can be distressing when your baby's arrival is not as you had envisioned or planned. These feelings are normal.

Talking about your disappointment with others can put your own experience in perspective. Reach out to other women you know who had cesarean sections and find out how they handled troublesome emotions. According to one sister, "None of my close friends delivered any of their babies by cesarean. We share everything with each other, but they just didn't know what I was feeling. I went to an online message board and read a bunch of birth stories posted by women who all had c-sections. The stories cheered me up because I no longer felt so alone. I eventually posted my own birth story so maybe another woman would read it and feel better. That's when I knew I was truly healed."

As time passes, you will probably feel differently about your childbirth experience. Contact your provider if feelings of disappointment or depression last longer than two weeks or become overwhelming. These emotions could signal postpartum depression.

Breastfeeding: The Healthiest Start

THE NUMBER OF plus-size women who breastfeed is well below the national average. While the reasons behind this unfortunate statistic are not entirely clear, choose to beat the odds. Breastfeed your baby. According to the National Women's Health Information Center, breastfeeding provides you and your baby with a staggering array of health benefits:

FOR BABY

- Breast milk is the perfect first food. Mother's milk contains the right amounts of fat, sugars, water, and protein needed for proper growth and development.
- Studies show breastfed infants, even those born with a high birth weight, are less likely to become overweight or obese as children. Breastfed babies grow exactly the way they should.
- Most babies find breast milk easier to digest than formula. This may mean fewer episodes of colic/fussiness and less spitting up.
- Breast milk contains antibodies to help protect infants from bacteria and viruses. Studies show that babies who are exclusively breastfed for six months or more are better at fighting off ear infections, diarrhea, and common respiratory illnesses. Breastfed babies require fewer doctors' visits.
- Because physical contact is so important to newborns, the close skin-to-skin contact of nursing helps your baby feel secure, warm and comforted.
- Preliminary studies indicate that infants who are *not* breastfed may have higher rates of sudden infant death syndrome (SIDS) in the first year of life, and higher rates of Type I and Type II diabetes, lymphoma, leukemia, Hodgkin's disease, overweight and obesity, high cholesterol, and asthma later in life.
- Breastfed babies score slightly higher on IQ tests.

FOR YOU

- Because you burn calories when you are breastfeeding (as many as 500 extra calories per day), shedding pounds and reaching a healthy weight might become a little easier.
- Breastfeeding lowers your risk for osteoporosis, breast cancer, and ovarian cancers.

- Breastfeeding triggers the release of oxytocin, a hormone that helps the uterus contract after birth. Oxytocin decreases blood loss and may shorten the amount of time you experience post-partum vaginal discharge (lochia).
- You will save money. Studies show women who breastfeed save over $1,000 during the first year of their baby's life simply because they don't need to buy formula and bottles!
- You will save time. There are no powders to measure and mix. There are no bottles to warm in the middle of the night. You can breastfeed anytime, anywhere.
- Breastfeeding enhances the mother–child bond. Women report increased self-confidence as mothers and deep feelings of closeness with their infants as a direct result of their choice to breastfeed.

Steps for Breastfeeding Success

BEFORE GIVING BIRTH

Learn as much as you can about breastfeeding. Find nursing role models by talking to plus-size women you know who are currently breastfeeding or who successfully nursed their children in the past. Go to a breastfeeding class offered through your hospital, provider's office, or local La Leche League chapter. Attend a breastfeeding support group even before your baby is born (usually offered by the same places). Joining a community of women who have all made the commitment to breastfeed can be powerful encouragement and motivation to stick with your choice to nurse.

BORN TO BREASTFEED

When do you start breastfeeding? If you are both physically up for it, you can nurse for the first time as soon as your baby is born. Babies are usually very alert in the first hour following birth and then drift off into a deep sleep. Amazing as this seems, newborns placed on their mothers' tummies right after birth instinctively root for their mother's breast, latch on, and start nursing—all by themselves!

Don't worry about what you will feed your baby—your body already has that all figured out. Until mature milk production begins, anywhere from two to four days after giving birth, your breasts produce *colostrum* for your baby to eat. This yellowish liquid contains important infection-fighting antibodies as well as protein and minerals.

You will know when mature milk production begins by the noticeably larger size and heavier feel of your breasts (large breasted women may only notice heavier breasts). Breast engorgement typically ends a few days after your milk comes in as milk production adjusts to your baby's needs. As mentioned before, the best relief for engorgement discomfort is breastfeeding your baby.

Nursing a Newborn

Breastfeeding your newborn presents a unique set of challenges. Unless you have nursed another child, both of you are doing something completely new. You are tired and probably sore from giving birth. If you had an epidural, your baby may also be groggy or even fussy.

Your tiny newborn requires extra gentle and supportive handling at all times. No matter what breastfeeding hold/position you use, you will need to make sure your newborn is correctly latched on to the breast. A proper latch can prevent nursing problems like sore nipples, low milk supply, and a baby who isn't gaining enough weight.

To help your baby establish a good latch, use your free hand to hold your breast just above the areola (darker area of skin around the nipple). Your hand should be held like the letter C, with the thumb resting on the top of the breast. Lightly compress the areola to better match up your breast to the shape of your baby's mouth. Brush your baby's lips with your nipple until your baby opens her mouth as big as a yawn. Center your nipple in your baby's mouth and gently pull your baby toward you.

Your baby's lips are rolled outward. Her chin is pressed into the breast while her nose lightly touches the breast. If your baby is latched correctly, her jaw noticeably moves up and down as she nurses and you will hear the reassuring sounds of a baby busily swallowing. In the early days it may take a few tries to achieve a successful latch.

Use the latch technique with any one of the following breastfeeding positions. The nursing holds we highlight offer plus-size women the best support and physical comfort for breastfeeding a newborn.

- **Crossover hold:** Sit up in bed or in a comfortable chair. Unwrap your baby down to only a diaper—this encourages wakefulness for eating and skin-to-skin contact with you promotes bonding. Use a nursing pillow or stack several pillows on your lap to support your baby's positioning as needed. If you start the feeding with your right breast, hold your baby with your left arm. Use your left hand to cradle the baby's neck and head. Lay your baby down on the pillow so he is turned and facing you, tummy to tummy. Your baby's head is positioned just in front of your right breast.

Hold your right breast with your right hand. The thumb and index finger should cup the breast in a C-shape just above the areola. Compress the areola to better match up your breast to the shape of your baby's mouth. Stimulate your baby to latch on. Nurse as long as your baby wants to, or until the breast is noticeably softer. Switch to left side if your baby is still hungry. Start with the left side the next time you nurse.

Women with larger breasts may feel more comfortable using the crossover hold because it provides more control. You will need to support your breast less and less as the two of you become more accustomed to nursing. This position may place pressure on your abdomen. If you are recovering from a c-section, ask a lactation consultant for help with this position (you can place pillow over your tummy to protect your healing incision).

- **Football hold:** For plus-size women who are large-breasted, the football or "clutch" hold allows for better visibility and control as your baby latches on to nurse. If you are recovering from a cesarean, there is no pressure on the abdomen in this position.

  As with the crossover hold, sit in a comfortable armchair. You can start with either the right or left breast (we are starting with the left in this example). Wedge a pillow between your left side and the chair. Cradling your baby's head with your left hand, tuck the baby under your left arm (your forearm provides support for baby's neck and back). Your baby now rests level with your waist and faces your left breast. You arm is held up by the wedged pillow.

  Hold your left breast with your right hand. Your thumb and index finger should cup the breast in a C-shape just above the areola. Compress the areola to better match up your breast to the shape of your baby's mouth. Stimulate the baby to latch on. Nurse as long as your baby wants to, or until the breast is noticeably softer. Switch to the right side if your baby is still hungry. Start with the right side the next time you nurse.

- **Side-lying:** This position is good for establishing first feedings if you are recovering from a cesarean section or if an episiotomy or sore perineum makes sitting up too uncomfortable.

Many women prefer to nurse in the side-lying position during late-night feedings.

You and your baby both lie on your sides, tummy to tummy. If recovering from a cesarean, have someone assist you in rolling over and make sure pillows are wedged behind your back for support. Your baby should be positioned level with your breast.

When lying on your right side, slightly lift your right breast with your left hand. Your thumb and index finger should cup the breast in a C-shape just above the areola. Compress the areola to better match up your breast to the shape of your baby's mouth. Stimulate the baby to latch on. Nurse as long as your baby wants to, or until the breast is noticeably softer. Switch sides and nurse your baby with your left breast if your baby is still hungry. Start with the left side the next time you nurse.

Establishing Your Milk Supply

Baby's first feedings trigger the complex hormonal reactions needed for mature milk production. According to some studies, plus-size women might be more likely than other women to encounter difficulties making breast milk. While you probably won't encounter serious problems, you should still learn everything you can about how to help your milk start flowing. The following steps will help you achieve breastfeeding success during those first few critical weeks.

- **Nurse early and often.** For best results in establishing your milk supply, start breastfeeding as soon as you can after birth. First nursing sessions may be brief but will gradually build in length, generally lasting anywhere from ten to forty-five minutes. Your newborn should nurse at least eight to twelve times during a 24-hour period. Emptying at least one breast at each feeding ensures you will have a constant and steady milk supply.

  During the first few days after birth, your baby may be very sleepy. If more than three hours have passed since the start of the last feeding, gently wake your baby up and encourage him to nurse. Undress your baby down to the diaper and rub his back to rouse him from sleep. Get into your preferred nursing position and encourage your baby to latch on. Skipped feedings may result in painful engorgement and an eventual slowdown in milk production.

- **Nurse on demand.** It's very simple: the more you breastfeed, the more milk you produce. Watch your baby for common feeding clues: nuzzling against your breast, sucking motions, and putting her hands to her mouth. Waiting until your baby cries out in hunger may backfire. A frantic baby may not calm down enough to nurse. Also, following a strict feeding schedule of nursing no more than once every three to four hours can seriously slow down milk production and deprive your baby of needed nourishment.

- **Room-in with your baby.** Make frequent breastfeeding easy and convenient by keeping your baby close to you during those first critical days and weeks. Once you give birth, unless health reasons dictate otherwise, your baby can room-in with you while you are at the hospital. When you come home, set up the crib or bassinet in your bedroom. Consider investing in a sidecar sleeper. Designed especially for breastfeeding mothers, a sidecar sleeper looks like a small crib with one side missing. It's secured flush against your bed and provides you with easier access to your baby for night feedings.

- **Limit visitors.** Most women need time and practice before they feel confident in their ability to breastfeed. Nursing is a learned art—for both of you! The best way to begin nursing is to create as relaxed and quiet an atmosphere as possible. Limit visitors to only those closest to you. If it makes you feel more comfortable, politely inform company they will need to leave once it's feeding time. As breastfeeding becomes more familiar, it should become much easier to have others around while you nurse.

- **Avoid supplemental bottle-feeding.** Giving your newborn bottles of formula or sugar water can wreak havoc with your milk supply. When your baby's demand to nurse drops because his appetite is satisfied elsewhere, milk production eventually slows down. While this is hopefully already hospital policy, let hospital staff know you are breastfeeding and request that no supplemental bottles or pacifiers be given to your newborn. If your newborn is unable to nurse for medical reasons, pump your colostrum/breast milk and use a feeding cup, supplemental nursing system, medicine dropper, or spoon to feed your baby. Pumping stimulates your breasts to continue producing milk. Most hospitals have electric pumps readily available.

Some experts believe introducing a bottle or pacifier before your baby has completely gotten the hang of breastfeeding can create "nipple confusion" and may cause your newborn to lose interest in nursing or even grow frustrated while at the breast. Rubber nipples and pacifiers encourage your baby to push the tongue forward and not fully open his mouth—the opposite of what is needed for a good nursing latch. Once you and your baby are comfortable with nursing, pumping bottles of expressed milk is a great way to let your partner or caregiver share in feeding times.

- **Recognize the signs of a well-fed baby.** A common worry among nursing mothers is whether or not their babies are getting enough nourishment through breast milk alone. Some easy-to-recognize signs that your breastfed baby is a well-fed baby include:

  - *Adequate weight gain:* Babies typically lose anywhere from 5 to 9 percent of their birth weight in the first few days following delivery. After your milk comes in, your baby should gain approximately 6 ounces per week. If you need reassurance that weight gain is on track, take your baby to the pediatrician's office for a weight check.
  - *Frequent diaper changes:* During the first few days after birth, your baby's bowel movements consist of *meconium*, sticky greenish-brown waste products that built up in the intestine before birth. Breastfeeding regularly helps rid the body of meconium and, by the end of the first week, stools should be soft, mustard colored, and seedy in appearance. From about the fourth day on, a well-nourished breastfed baby should have three or more bowel movements a day (usually six or more). Likewise, approximately eight wet-diaper changes a day provide a good sign your baby is well-hydrated and getting enough to eat.
  - *Sights and sounds of a satisfied eater:* Most newborns nurse in spurts, suckling vigorously for a few minutes, resting, and then beginning again. You will notice strong, rhythmic motions in your baby's cheeks during nursing. A satisfied baby usually falls asleep or becomes very

drowsy by the end of the feeding. If your baby makes clicking noises or you notice her cheeks are dimpled while nursing, these are signs your baby is not latched on properly and is probably not getting enough to eat. Reposition your baby as needed to achieve a good latch.

- **Take care of your breasts.** It's normal to feel nipple tenderness during the first few days of nursing. Because an improper nursing latch is usually the cause of most nipple discomfort, pay special attention to baby's positioning at the breast. Make sure your baby is not clamped on the nipple, but has almost the entire areola in her mouth. If your breasts are engorged after your milk comes in, achieve a proper latch by first expressing milk for a few minutes (pump or manually) to soften the areola.

  Keep your nipples healthy by allowing your breasts to air-dry for about ten minutes after the nursing session ends. Avoid wearing nursing pads with moisture-trapping plastic liners. Soap or shampoo can dry out or irritate already tender nipples. Allow the areola and nipples to clean themselves with their own naturally occurring oils.

  Some women find relief for sore nipples by applying purified lanolin cream (Lanisoh or Pur Lan). These creams may also promote healing in dry, cracked nipples. A drop of breast milk gently rubbed into your nipples may also speed healing. Call your provider if you have a red, sore or painful area on your breast, you have painful engorgement, a fever, or you feel achy. These may be signs of a breast infection (*mastitis*).

- **Dress the part.** Wearing a nursing bra provides support for larger, heavier breasts and helps prevent back strain. Fold-down flaps make the frequent nursing schedule of a newborn convenient at home or on the go. Try to find cotton bras for better "breathability."

  Adding a few nursing tops to your wardrobe means you will be able to discreetly nurse your baby no matter when or where the need arises—perfect for that eventual day when you can no longer hold back the throng of visitors trying to catch a glimpse of your new arrival. Any kind of shirt that can be lifted up or unbuttoned in the front can turn into a nursing top. Try a nursing cape or poncho if it makes you more comfortable about nursing in public. See Resources for retailers who carry plus-size nursing clothing, bras, and other nursing-related products.

- **Keep eating right!** The balanced diet you followed during pregnancy is still important now that you are nursing. Fill your menu with plenty of fruits and vegetables, fish, chicken, whole grains, milk, and healthy fats. Eat salmon and omega-3 fortified eggs for your baby's brain and eye development. Healthy meals and snacks boost your energy levels during the exhausting early weeks of motherhood. Eating nutrient-rich foods replenishes the vitamins and minerals used to make breast milk.

  To prevent any deficiencies, keep taking your daily prenatal vitamin. If you are vegan, take a separate B_{12} supplement to ensure your breast milk contains adequate levels. You should also drink about 8 to 10 cups of water each day to keep up fluid levels needed for milk production. Rule of thumb: keep a glass of water, vegetable juice, seltzer, or iced herbal tea next to you when you sit down to nurse.

  Some food ingredients can pass to your baby through your breast milk. Spicy foods, chocolate, and caffeine (more than 1 or 2 cups of coffee per day) may cause your baby to become irritable after nursing. You may need to eliminate or cut back on these foods for the first few months of breastfeeding. While it might sound like the only thing that will zap your exhaustion, hold off on that triple espresso chocolate latte. A baby who is less irritable after feeding is more likely to fall asleep—giving you time to catch up on your own much-needed rest.

  Finally, breastfeeding is helpful in your postpartum efforts to lose weight. Losing 1 pound per week is a healthy weight-loss goal for a nursing woman. Use the scale as your guide for how many calories you should consume each day. Don't be surprised if you are able to eat a little more than you usually would on a typical weight-loss diet—making breast milk is helping you burn an extra 500 extra calories per day.

- **Get help from a certified lactation specialist.** Most hospitals have lactation specialists on staff, often RNs who are specially trained to teach and troubleshoot breastfeeding techniques. If you find early attempts to breastfeed painful, your baby won't latch on properly, or nursing just doesn't seem to be working out for either you or your baby, ask to consult with a lactation specialist while you are in the hospital.

The lactation specialist will observe you nurse your baby and then offer encouraging support and practical advice for proper latch on and positioning. This person wants you to succeed at breastfeeding and will offer a variety of suggestions until you find what works best for you.

Check with your hospital, provider's office, or your baby's pediatrician (many have lactation consultants on staff) to see what lactation services are available in your area. Some lactation specialists even make house calls!

Even if you don't require any help in the beginning, you can contact a lactation specialist with any questions that pop up in the months ahead. Many nursing mothers who return to work have questions about how to successfully combine work and breastfeeding. Lactation specialists can help you with pump rentals and provide information about how to keep your milk flowing long after your maternity leave has ended.

Have patience as you and your baby get to know each other. Don't give up! Each time you nurse think about the numerous benefits you are giving your baby—and yourself. If you get off to a rocky start, don't delay in getting help from a lactation specialist. Connect with other nursing women for support, even if all this means is calling your sister long-distance and asking how she handled sore nipples.

Keep breastfeeding your baby. One of motherhood's finest moments is gazing down at your busily nursing infant, realizing that your nourishment is solely responsible for fueling this healthy, thriving little person.

Postpartum Depression

AS MANY AS 80 percent of all new mothers experience moodiness, mild anxiety, depression, and/or feelings of sadness sometime during the first week or so after giving birth. Called the "baby blues," these troubling emotions are due in part to the sudden drop in certain hormones following delivery (estrogen and progesterone). The blues are temporary and manageable for most women and usually disappear as hormone levels stabilize.

When emotional symptoms are severe, continue beyond the second postpartum week, or start anytime during the first year after giving birth and last longer than two weeks, it may mean you have developed postpartum depression. Approximately 10 percent of all new mothers encounter this mood disorder. Are you at risk for postpartum depression? Women are more likely to experience postpartum depression if they were depressed before or during pregnancy, had a difficult/ complicated pregnancy or delivery, have family members who suffer from depression, or are under a great deal of emotional stress. Statistically, more plus-size women suffer from depression.

Contact your provider immediately if you notice any of these symptoms:

- "Baby blues" lasting longer than two weeks
- Deep depression or anger appearing anytime within a year from your baby's birth
- Troubling feelings of sadness, doubt, guilt, or hopelessness that grow progressively worse and hamper your ability to take good care of yourself and your baby
- Sleeplessness, even when you are exhausted
- Sleeping most of the time; not being able to wake up to care for your baby
- Overeating or eating very little
- Panic attacks and constant worry
- Lack of interest in your baby or family
- Thoughts of harming yourself or your baby. In this situation, do not hesitate to call 911.

Managing Your Postpartum Depression

- **Don't hide your feelings.** Like many women, you may be tempted to deny your feelings of depression because you fear it makes you look like a failure. Nothing could be further from the truth. Confronting depression and asking for help takes courage. A successful mother is a woman who doesn't let anything stand in the way of taking good care of her baby—or herself. Confide your feelings in your partner and contact your provider. Get the help you deserve.
- **Rest.** Fatigue and exhaustion can intensify postpartum depression (extreme tiredness may even help trigger the disorder). In addition to your partner's assistance, ask close friends and family to help you out around the house so you can catch up on your sleep.
- **Exercise.** Physical activity is a natural mood lifter. As soon as

you recover from childbirth and get your provider's approval, start going for a brisk walk every day.

- **Find support.** Call Depression After Delivery (1-800-944-4PPD), a national referral service to help you locate local support groups. See Resources, for recommended postpartum support Web sites.
- **Have your thyroid checked.** Levels of thyroid hormones may also drop after giving birth. The thyroid is a small gland in the neck that helps regulate your metabolism. Low thyroid levels can cause symptoms of depression including depressed mood, irritability, fatigue, difficulty concentrating, sleep problems, and weight gain. A simple blood test can tell if a thyroid problem is causing your depression. Your provider may prescribe a thyroid medicine to treat this condition.
- **Investigate treatment options.** Depending on the severity of your depression, your provider may suggest a variety of therapies to treat your condition, including talking to a counselor/therapist or using medication. For breastfeeding women, taking any kind of medicine is cause for concern because small amounts can enter your breast milk. Antidepressants such as Zoloft (sertaline) are generally considered safe for nursing mothers.

Postpartum Weight Loss and Exercise

I remember coming home from the hospital after having Avery. My husband asked what I wanted for dinner. Without even thinking about it, I requested my favorite dish during pregnancy: whole-grain couscous with chicken and vegetables. As we were eating, my husband and I talked about how we couldn't wait until our first walk together as a family. That's when it finally clicked. For the past nine months, a healthy, active lifestyle had gradually become second nature.

—ALICIA, age 24

IF YOU, LIKE so many other plus-size women, once yo-yo dieted your way up the scale, the topic of weight loss may bring back bad memories of restricting food intake to three cans of diet drink a day or eating only steak, bacon, and cheese for weeks. Over the past nine months you have hopefully practiced the basics of healthy eating. Don't get back on the diet roller coaster. Make good food choices a permanent part your postpartum life. As much as the diet industry wants you to believe otherwise, eating a healthy, balanced diet, and regularly exercising is the perfect recipe for permanently shedding excess pounds.

Successful postpartum weight loss is a gradual process. We offer the following suggestions to help you reach a healthier weight:

- **Determine your ideal weight.** How much should you weigh? How much weight do you need to lose? Flip back to the first chapter and look at the Body Mass Index chart. You used it before to determine your prepregnancy BMI. Now find out how much you need to weigh in order to fall within the "normal BMI" range for your height (a BMI between 20 and 25). This is your goal weight range. Calculate the number of pounds you will need to lose before reaching a normal BMI.

- **Wait until you are ready.** Your body needs time to recuperate from pregnancy and childbirth. Experts recommend not starting any weight-loss diet until at least six weeks following childbirth. Discuss weight-loss plans with your provider at your postpartum checkup. Your provider can determine if your body is ready to resume physical activity and give you feedback about the weight-loss diet you have chosen to follow. Until you meet with your provider, your best bet is to stick with your healthy prenatal menu plan.

- **Take it slow.** During the first few days and weeks after birth you naturally lose many of the pounds you put on during pregnancy (as many as 15 pounds or more). After this initial weight loss tapers off, many women may be tempted to drastically cut calories to quickly lose even more weight. As we all already know from years of dieting, this scheme rarely works.

  Make your goal gradual weight loss—approximately 1 to 2 pounds per week. Plan your diet around the same food groups and serving sizes described in chapter 5, "Prenatal Nutrition." To cut enough calories for weight loss, choose low-fat instead of whole milk, fill your plate with lots of high-fiber vegetables, and eliminate all sugary, processed foods from your diet. Exercising thirty minutes a day will burn excess calories and enhance your weight-loss efforts. As you did during pregnancy, let the scale be your guide. If your weight stays the same or goes up, cut more calories and increase your physical activity.

- **Consult with a nutritionist.** You may have met with a nutritionist during pregnancy to create a balanced prenatal menu plan. Meet with the nutritionist again, this time to construct a healthy postpartum weight-loss diet. You may be surprised to find that what you ate during pregnancy and what you should eat now to lose weight are not very different. A nutritionist will work with you to determine the precise number of calories you should consume each day to reach your gradual weight-loss goals.

- **Resume your exercise routine.** Once you get the green light from your provider to start exercising, don't necessarily expect to pick up where you left off before giving birth. If during pregnancy you had built up to an hour-long power walk, you may be only able to walk for ten to twenty minutes before you become exhausted. This is normal. Keep going out for brief walks (or a shorter form of your favorite exercise) and slowly build up from there. Contact your provider if you feel dizzy or faint while exercising.

- **Consider joining a weight-loss support group.** Check into whether or not your hospital offers a weight-loss support group. Larger hospitals may offer groups specifically for postpartum women. To deal with emotional issues related to food, attend an Overeaters Anonymous meeting. Joining Weight Watchers may provide the structure and positive encouragement you need to stick with your weight-loss program. There are many weight-loss support options available, choose the one that best fits your needs.

- **Remind yourself why you are doing this.** Your intense desire to have a healthy baby helped you successfully change your eating and exercise habits during pregnancy. Stay motivated. Losing your extra weight and lowering your BMI to within normal range provides you with countless health benefits. You will feel more energetic. You will be less likely to encounter such health problems as Type II diabetes and heart disease. You won't need to worry as much about complications in future pregnancies. You will cut your risk for breast, ovarian, and many other types of cancer. You will live longer. You will become a positive role model to your child.

It's always a nice bonus to fit into the jeans you wore in high school, but knowing that losing weight makes it more likely for your children to grow up into healthy adults (and for you to more richly share in their lives) supplies the deep motivation needed to sustain your weight-loss efforts over the long-haul. Write down all the reasons you have for losing weight and post it prominently on the fridge. Don't forget why your healthy lifestyle is so important!

Growing a Healthy Family

I was pregnant just as the media started paying more attention to America's weight problem, in particular childhood obesity. As I watched news segments and read newspaper articles about childhood obesity, I began to identify the reasons why I had become overweight in my early teens. All the bad habits that commonly lead to childhood obesity—too much TV, not enough exercise, eating too much fast food instead of home cooking—were clearly present during my younger years.

My heart broke for the kids featured on the news broadcasts because I saw myself in each of their faces. I vowed that things would be very different for my baby. All I needed to do was find out the answer to one very big question: How do I guide my daughter in creating a healthy, active lifestyle when I never experienced one growing up?

—ANDREA, age 24

YOU WATCHED WHAT you ate, you exercised during pregnancy—you changed your life to give your baby the best chance possible at being born healthy. Decisions you make now and how you raise your child in the months and years ahead are equally important. The family lifestyle you and your partner create will leave a lasting impression on your child's life. Your child will reflect your choices as a parent.

The current childhood obesity epidemic underscores how important it is for parents to make good choices about nutrition and physical activity. More then 15 percent of children age six to eleven are obese, and more than 10 percent of all two- to five-year-olds! Childhood obesity is linked with more time spent watching TV and playing video games, less outdoor play, fewer opportunities for physical education in school, diets high in processed foods, and too much eating out. Studies show overweight and obese parents are more likely to raise children who will themselves encounter weight problems.

You learned everything you needed to know in order to have a successful plus-size pregnancy. Devote that same energy to giving your child a healthy life, starting from the first moment you hold your newborn in your arms. Practical steps for creating a fit, happy, and healthy family include:

- **Breastfeed your baby.** In the middle of the childhood obesity crisis is some very positive news. According to recent studies, breastfed babies are as much as 30 percent less likely to become obese as children. The longer a baby is breastfed, the lower the risk for encountering weight problems. To reap the full benefits of breastfeeding, the American Academy of Pediatricians recommends exclusively breastfeeding for the first six months of life and after solids have been introduced, continuing to breastfeed until at least your baby's first birthday.
- **Lead by example.** Dedicate yourself to healthy eating and physical activity. When you eat nutritious foods, you are a better role model for your child's own diet. As you lose weight and exercise, you will probably find yourself more energetic and more willing to do all those crazy, silly things that babies seem to love. Whether you have a son or daughter, you are your baby's primary role model from the very beginning. Your healthy lifestyle does not go unnoticed by your child.

  As one sister reported about her healthier eating and exercise habits, "I see my four-month-old daughter watching me when I grab a shiny apple out of the fruit bowl. The other day she even said something that sounded like 'apple'! It might seem really simple, but I know this is a really important start toward a healthy future for both of us!"
- **Avoid exposing your child to "educational" TV shows, videos, and DVDs.** They promise to provide intellectual stimulation and educational fun, but programs geared for infants and toddlers also give your baby a head start on watching too much TV—one of the leading causes of childhood obesity. In general, young children should not watch any TV.

  Instead of allowing your baby to sit passively in front of the TV, help your little one find delight and stimulation in his own world. Hang some wind chimes on the porch. Sit outside together on a breezy day and listen to the gentle chiming melodies. Actually feeling the wind and then seeing the chimes blow about and ring can make powerful connections in your baby's brain about the way the world works. Install a window-mounted bird feeder and watch your baby gurgle in delight each time a new bird stops by for a snack. Read to your baby. Show him all the excitement and pleasure to be found between the pages of a book. Go to the park and watch the autumn leaves fall from the trees. Pick up the ones you both watched float to the ground. Examine every tiny vein and nuance of color. This is a very different experience from watching a video about the changing seasons.

If plopping your baby in front of the TV is the only way for you to get some free time during the day, consider other TV-free options. Are there other mothers, fathers, or caregivers in your apartment building or neighborhood interested in forming a babysitting exchange? Members could take turns watching each other's children so each parent has a few hours a week for "alone time." Establish "no TV" ground rules during the swaps. Another alternative is to advertise for a mother's helper or enlist your family members to help you out. While they play with the baby, you are free to take that really long, hot shower you have been fantasizing about.

- **Advocate for your baby's good nutrition.** When your baby starts solids (usually recommended around six months), always check the ingredient label before buying baby food. Jarred baby food should only contain pureed fruits and vegetables (and possibly water). Avoid brands with added sugar or salt. As soon as your baby is able to eat them, switch to mashed bananas and other simple foods you prepare fresh yourself. Start with whole instead of processed grains when choosing baby cereals. Some brands now market brown rice cereal.

When it comes to snacks, skip the baby/toddler cereal bars entirely or carefully read labels before purchasing. As of 2006, trans fats (partially hydrogenated oils) must be listed on food labels. Many companies have reformulated their recipes and omitted trans fats from cereal bars and toddler snacks. Some have not. Also, leaving out trans fats still doesn't make processed snack food for babies and toddlers a healthy food choice. Ingredients such as high-fructose corn syrup, chemical preservatives, and too much salt/sodium still remain. If you need an on-the-go snack, try sliced fruit, bananas, a bagful of Cheerios, or make bran or whole-grain blueberry muffins from scratch (substitute your baby's favorite fresh fruit). Muffins don't take much time to prepare, contain relatively inexpensive ingredients, make your house smell delicious, and are a portable, healthier snack choice for your baby.

By your baby's first birthday, your freshly minted toddler will be able to eat the same foods as the rest of the family—just leave out any heavy spices, and mash or cut food into small pieces.

While your toddler will no doubt be very picky and hesitant to try new foods, keep offering nutritious, balanced meals. Avoid the quick fix of fast-food chicken nuggets with dipping sauce and french fries (french-fried potatoes are the most commonly eaten vegetable by young children); these foods train your toddler's taste buds to like greasy, sweet, and salty flavors. In general, avoid bringing your child to fast-food restaurants.

Remain persistent in offering healthy meals and snacks. It may take as many as ten times before your toddler will try a new food, but it will eventually happen. Read some of the many books devoted to toddler-friendly meal planning (see Resources). Use tried-and-true tricks parents have relied on for years to win over resistant eaters: arrange cut fruit to resemble a happy face, spell out your baby's name with peas, call mashed potatoes "cloud nibbles." As one mother says, "When it comes to getting my toddler to eat what I want her to eat, it's all about the marketing!"

If your baby with the voracious appetite becomes a toddler who just won't eat very much, it's probably not time to worry. Toddlers generally have smaller appetites because they are not growing as fast as they did during their first year of life. If your toddler is active, healthy, and growing and developing normally, then she is most likely getting plenty to eat.

- **Take parenting classes.** To equip parents with the necessary tools to raise healthy, active children, many hospitals and large pediatric practices now offer parenting classes that go beyond how to diaper, burp, and bathe a newborn. You may be able to attend seminars and classes on topics ranging from breast-feeding support, toddler and school-age nutrition, balancing work and parenting, healthy family cooking, and even post-partum yoga classes for you *and* your baby (usually when your baby is at least six weeks old). Call your pediatrician's office or hospital's community outreach center to find out more about educational opportunities in your area.

- **Join a "new mother" support group.** Like parenting classes, new mother support groups (as well as those for a "new dad" and "new parents") are usually offered through a pediatrician's office or the hospital. Groups are facilitated by a nurse, pediatrician, or postpartum counselor. In addition to discussing your most pressing postpartum concerns and questions, support groups are good places to meet other women doing everything they can to get their new families off to a success-ful start. Maybe you will encounter a mom who lives nearby and wants to meet up at the park for an outing. Maybe another mom is starting a morning power-walking club—babies wel-come. Churches and other religious organizations sometimes sponsor parenting support groups. La Leche League offers groups specifically for new mothers who are nursing.

- **Increase physical activity in your family's daily life.** Become a regular at the park playground. As soon as your baby is able to sit up (around six months), he can use the infant swings and you can hold him as he goes down one of the smaller slides. In addition to the good times you will share together as a family on these park outings, from a very early age your baby will see lots of other kids running around having a great time.

  Join the YMCA or other family-oriented fitness center. Some parent-child movement and swim classes are geared for babies as young as six weeks old. Not only will you introduce your baby to the fun of physical activity, you will meet other like-minded families through these classes.

  Of course, one of the easiest ways to jump-start a physically active family lifestyle is to simply go for a daily family walk together. Start as soon as you have physically recovered from birth. Skip the stroller as much as possible, and use a front car-rier or sling to "wear your baby" while you walk (see "Resources" for carriers and slings made specifically for plus-size women). Some advantages to a carrier: you get a better workout, your baby gets to see the world from your point of view, and walking motions may soothe a cranky baby.

- **Go outside.** From the 1970s to the present, children have spent less and less time playing outside. At the same time, childhood obesity rates have gone up. Make being outdoors a natural part of your child's life from the very beginning. Take your crawling baby to the park and let her creep after the squir-rels. Let your wobbly toddler learn to walk among the soft pine needles at the nearby state forest. Sit outside together on a warm summer night and count the stars or watch the fireflies dance overhead.

  Going on vacation? Plan your family trips around outdoor activities. Many summer camps and campgrounds offer fam-ily programs with activities for both young children and parents.

Spend the day at the petting zoo or a working farm that encourages visitors. Go on a walking tour if you vacation in a large city or spend a relaxing day at the beach building sandcastles.

- **Find quality child care.** If you are planning on returning to work, seek out child care that reflects your values. While visiting in-home day-care providers and day-care centers, find out the answers to all the usual questions—provider-to-child ratio, available hours, rates—but also evaluate day-care sites for how helpful they will be in helping you raise an active, healthy child. Find out up front what foods are offered and how much age-appropriate physical activity is scheduled each day. Is there a fenced-in outdoor play area with lots of safe equipment? Especially for in-home care providers: is the TV ever on during the day? If so, what is the provider's policy (one hour on rainy days, or unlimited access)?

  If you will continue to breastfeed after you return to work, is the provider/center comfortable with you stopping by on your lunch break to nurse? Will the provider give your baby a bottle of pumped milk *first* and only supplement with formula if absolutely necessary? What kind of solid food is served? Does the provider use whole-grain cereal? Make sure the toddler menu offers fresh fruits and vegetables and the provider/center does not use foods with trans fats and high-fructose corn syrup. If you generally like the provider or center—just not the menu—request that you provide your child's own food (this is already the policy for many providers/centers).

Don't Forget What is Most Important.

SOME OF THE best advice for growing a healthy family? No matter how you spend time together as a family, have fun! Remember the daydreams you had about all the wonderful things you would do together once your baby arrived? Make your dreams into reality! Enjoying the time you spend with each other is what a great family life is all about.

GLOSSARY

ACE INHIBITORS: a type of medication used for the treatment of hypertension that should not be used during pregnancy

AFP (ALPHA-FETOPROTEIN) TESTING: one of a series of markers found in the blood of pregnant women; used to determine the risk that the unborn baby may have certain abnormalities

AFTERPAINS: uterine contractions after the delivery of the placenta

AMNIOTIC FLUID: fluid surrounding the baby while in the uterus

AREOLAE: darker skin around the nipples of the human breasts

AUSCULTATION: the act of listening to sounds within organs, such as a fetus's heartbeat

BASAL BODY TEMPERATURE: core body temperature in a resting state

BLASTOCYST: a name for the collection of cells that appear the first week after fertilization of an egg

BODY MASS INDEX (BMI): a ratio of weight to height that is used to make estimates of health risks

BRAXTON-HICKS CONTRACTIONS: uterine contractions of the pregnant uterus that do not lead to changes in the cervix

CERTIFIED NURSE MIDWIFE (CNM): a nurse with specialized training who is certified through the American College of Nurse Midwives in the care of women and the delivery of their babies

CESAREAN SECTION, C-SECTION: the method of delivering a baby through an abdominal incision

CHRONIC HYPERTENSION: high blood pressure that has been persistent

CLOMIPHINE CITRATE (CLOMID): a medication that has been used to stimulate ovulation in certain women with infertility

COLOSTRUM: the first milk produced after delivery and often in the weeks prior to labor

CROWNING: the point in the second stage of labor when the vulva is stretched tightly around the top of the soon-to-be born baby's head

DIASTOLIC PRESSURE: the blood pressure in your arteries between heart beats

DILATE: open

DOPPLER ULTRASOUND: high frequency sound waves used to create an image or a sound

DOULA: a specialized labor support person

DYSTOCIA: difficult delivery

EDEMA: swelling

EFFACE: shortening and thinning

EMBRYO: the developing baby from conception until the end of the second month

ENDOTHELIAL CELLS: a thin layer of cells lining blood vessels and other structures

ENGORGEMENT: swelling, usually used in referring to breasts as they fill with milk

EPIDURAL: a type of regional anesthesia that provides pain relief from the waist down

ESSENTIAL FATS: fats that cannot be made by the human body

FALLOPIAN TUBE: the structure that allows the human egg to pass from the ovary into the uterus

FETOSCOPE: a device for listening to the unborn baby's heart beat

FETUS: the unborn baby from 9 weeks gestation until delivery

FOLATE/FOLIC ACID: a B vitamin important in the development of the fetus, especially important in the formation of the neural neural tube; may also play a role in the prevention of adult heart disease

FSH (FOLLICLE STIMULATING HORMONE): a hormone made by the pituitary gland which regulates the hormones associated with ovulation

FUNDAL HEIGHT: the measurement of the growing pregnant uterus from the pubic bone to the top of the uterus (fundus)

GESTATIONAL AGE: the number of weeks of pregnancy dating from last menstrual period (in an idealized 28-day cycle)

GESTATIONAL DIABETES: a difficulty in the metabolism of sugar which appears during pregnancy

GESTATIONAL HYPERTENSION: high blood pressure that appears during pregnancy

GLUCOMETER: a device for measuring blood sugar levels

GLUCOSE CHALLENGE TEST: a blood test done 1 hour after a 50 gram oral dose of glucose is given

GLUCOSE TOLERANCE TEST: a 3-hour series of blood tests done in the fasting state and after a 100 gram oral dose of glucose is given

GLYCEMIC INDEX: a measure of how different foods affect a person's blood sugar

HDL (HIGH-DENSITY LIPOPROTEIN): a type of cholesterol which is considered beneficial

HEME-IRON: iron bound to blood cells

HEMORRHOIDS: varicose veins of the anal area, may become inflamed and painful

HUMALOG: fast-acting insulin

HYPNOBIRTHING: a relaxation/self-hypnotic technique used for the management of pain associated with labor

HYPOGLYCEMIA: low blood sugar

IN VITRO FERTILIZATION (IVF): fertilization of a mammalian egg outside of the human body prior to being returned to the uterus

INDUCED LABOR/INDUCTION: labor that is brought on by artificial means

INSULIN: a hormone important in the regulation of blood sugar levels

INTRAABDOMINAL: inside the abdomen

INTRAUTERINE GROWTH RESTRICTION (IUGR): unusually small babies for the length of pregnancy

IRON-DEFICIENCY ANEMIA: low blood count associated with inadequate iron intake

ISCHIAL SPINES: landmarks in the human pelvis used to measure the baby's downward progress

LANUGO: fine, soft hair

LMP: last menstrual period, used in arriving at a due date in a pregnant woman

LDL (LOW-DENSITY LIPOPROTEIN): a type of cholesterol that, if elevated, is considering unhealthy

LH (LUTEINIZING HORMONE): a hormone made by the pituitary that regulates ovulation

LIGHTENING: when the baby settles lower in the pelvis, usually in the last month of pregnancy

LISTERIA: a bacterium that can contaminate food and cause disease especially dangerous to the unborn baby

LOCHIA: bloody vaginal discharge after the birth of a baby

MACROSOMIA: large size as it refers to a baby, usually weighing more than 10 pounds.

MASTITIS: infection of the breast

MECONIUM: early stool of the newborn

MORNING SICKNESS: nausea and sometimes vomiting associated with pregnancy

NEURAL TUBE: a structure in the fetus which will become the central nervous system (brain and spinal cord)

NEURAL TUBE DEFECTS (NTDs): abnormalities in development of the spinal cord and brain

NICU: neonatal intensive care unit, a unit in the hospital which cares for ill or premature babies

NONSTRESS TESTS (NSTs): special fetal testing which monitors a baby's heart rate prior to labor and birth

NPH: intermediate-acting insulin

OMEGA-3 FATTY ACIDS: an essential fatty acid

OXYTOXIN: a natural hormone important in the initiation and progress of labor

PALPATE: to feel

PERINATOLOGIST: an obstetrician specializing in the care of high risk pregnant patients

PERINEUM: the area between the vagina and anus

PITOCIN: a synthetic form of the hormone oxytocin

PLACENTA PREVIA: a placenta (afterbirth) which covers the cervix completely

POLYCYSTIC OVARY SYNDROME (PCOS): a condition characterized by irregular, or no, ovulation, abnormal hair growth and other hormonal abnormalities, often associated with small cysts in the ovaries

PREECLAMPSIA: hypertension in pregnancy associated with protein in the urine and usually swelling of the feet

PROSTAGLANDIN: a hormone important in the preparation of the cervix for labor

PROTEINURIA: protein in the urine

QUICKENING: first perceptible movements of a fetus

RECOMMENDED DAILY ALLOWANCE (RDA): recommendations of the USDA for the daily intake of certain nutrients

SHOULDER DYSTOCIA: difficulty in the delivery of the baby's shoulders once the head has emerged from the vagina

SHOW: a blood-tinged discharge from the vagina associated with loss of the mucous plug or labor

SITZ BATH: a device used for soaking the perineum in a small amount of water

SLEEP APNEA: a period during sleep when breathing temporarily stops for a short period of time

SONOGRAM: a technique using high frequency sound waves to view internal organs

SPINA BIFIDA: a neural tube defect of the spine and spinal cord

SYSTOLIC PRESSURE: the blood pressure in your arteries as your heart is contracting

TELEMETRY: a method of monitoring your baby's heartbeat when you are not physically attached to a fetal monitor

TOXEMIA: see preeclampsia

TOXOPLASMOSIS: an infection that is transmitted in raw meat and cat feces that can be harmful to your unborn baby

TRANS FATS/TRANS FATTY ACID: fats that have been chemically altered by adding hydrogen atoms, making the fats more hydrogenated

TRANSDUCER: a device used to change one form of energy to another, in obstetrics, can be used to convert ultrasound to images or sound

TRIMESTER: a 3-month period of time during pregnancy

TYPE I DIABETES: a disease characterized by the body's inability to make insulin resulting in abnormally high blood sugars

TYPE II DIABETES: a type of diabetes where the body is unable to make enough insulin to meet demands

ULTRASOUND: high frequency sound waves

VBAC: vaginal birth after cesarean section

VENA CAVA: the large vein which carries blood from your body back to the heart

RESOURCES

IF YOU WANT to learn more about plus-size pregnancy as well as other topics we've addressed in the previous pages, the following resource list highlights the best and most relevant contacts, books, and Web sites.

Plus-Size Pregnancy/Support

The Plus-Size Pregnancy Web Site
www.plus-size-pregnancy.org
Created by a plus-size mom who is also a midwife, the site provides detailed and well-researched information about everything from plus-size maternity clothes to gestational diabetes. Check out the inspirational plus-size birth stories!

Plus-Sized and Pregnant
www.bbs.babycenter.com/board/pregnancy/8404
High-traffic message board where plus-size moms-to-be share advice, support, and friendship.

Overweight & Pregnant Support (OPSS)
www.fertilityplus.org/bbw/opss.html
High-volume listserv dedicated to discussing weight-related pregnancy issues, especially plus-size pregnancy after infertility. Intended primarily for women who are at least 50 pounds overweight.

Plus-Size Maternity/
Nursing Clothes and Nursing Bras

Retail Stores

Fashion Bug
www.fashionbug.charmingshoppes.com
Trendy plus-size maternity clothes available in sizes 1X to 3X.
   Check Web site for store locator or to buy clothes online.

Motherhood Maternity
1-800-4mom2be (1-800-466-6223)
www.motherhood.com
Retail locations nationwide carry plus-sizes 1X through 3X.
   Call for a store near you.

Old Navy
www.oldnavy.com
Maternity clothes stocked up to size 20. Check their Web site for
   store locator.

Target Stores
www.target.com
Most maternity clothes are available up to XXL (size 20 for
   pants). More styles are available on the Web site than in-store.
   Call 1-800-440-0680 for closest retail location.

Online/Catalog Only

Baby Becoming Plus-Size Maternity
www.babybecoming.com
Plus-size maternity and nursing clothing in sizes 1X through 6X
   (including pantyhose). Also carries slings and nursing pillows
   suitable for plus-size bodies.

Decent Exposures
www.decentexposures.com
Offers cotton and cotton/lycra blend nursing bras in sizes up
   through 54L. Organic cotton and velour bras available. Carries
   panties and some maternity separates up through size 4X. Call
   1-800-524-4949 to request catalog.

Jake & Me Maternity & Nursing Clothing
www.jakeandme.com
Tall and petite clothing through size 4X.

JC Penney
www.jcpenney.com
Stop by the store to pick up the maternity catalog or shop online.
JC Penney offers sizes through 3X. Good selection of casual
separates and career wear. Some dressier outfits available for
special occasions.

Lane Bryant Catalog
www.lbcatalog.com
Offers basic maternity wardrobe separates in sizes 14 through 32
(including plus-size maternity swimsuits). Call 1-800-228-
3120 for a free print catalog.

Make Your Own Nursing Tee
http://web.winco.net/~sbcortlu/makeyourowntee.htm
Provides simple instructions to turn one of your own T-shirts into
a nursing top. Minimal sewing skills required.

Maternity for Less
www.maternity4less.com
In addition to a nice variety of reasonably priced "basics," you will
find plus-size maternity clothes suitable for dressier occasions.
Sizes through 3X.

Motherwear
www.motherwear.com
Specializes in clothing for breastfeeding women. Selected tops,
dresses, and sleepwear in sizes 2X through 4X. Nursing bras in
sizes through 50J. Call 1-800-633-0303 for a free print catalog.

Pickles and Ice Cream Plus-Size Maternity Fashions
www.plusmaternity.com
Waist, bust, hip, and length measurements for each item are
given in order for shoppers to more easily purchase the correct
size.

Baby Carriers

Over-the-Shoulder Baby Carrier
1-800-637-9426
www.babyholder.com
Beautifully made slings. Size L fits parents from 140 to 250
pounds. Company will also custom-sew XL, XXL, or XXXL
slings for an additional $10.

Baby Trekker
1-800-665-3957
www.babytrekker.com
These rugged front carriers are designed with a waist support to
more evenly distribute baby's weight. Converts to backpack
carrier. Size L, "Extra Roomy Trekker," fits up to a 50-inch
waist. Padded for comfort.

The Baby Wearer: Tips for Plus-Size Babywearing
www.thebabywearer.com/articles/WhatToO/PlusSizes.htm
A plus-size mom reports on how well different slings and front
carriers work for larger women.

Body Image/ Body Acceptance

Marcia Hutchinson, 200 Ways to Love the Body You Have (Freedom,
CA: Crossing Press, 1999).
Promotes body acceptance through guided imagery, relaxation,
and journaling techniques.

Body Positive
www.bodypositive.org
Tips and advice for feeling good about your body—no matter how
much you weigh.

Health at Any Size Web Ring
http://d.webring.com/hub?ring=anysize
Links to numerous body/size acceptance Web sites.

Breastfeeding

American Academy of Pediatricians
www.aap.org/healthtopics/breastfeeding.cfm
This Web site includes extensive information about breastfeeding as well as the latest guidelines and recommendations.

Breastfeeding.com
www.breastfeeding.com
With an active community message board and an extensive question and answer section (and much more), this is the ultimate Web site for nursing mothers.

Breastfeeding for African American Women
www.4woman.gov/pub/BF.AA.pdf
Breastfeeding advice tailored to fit the needs of African-American women, in a 36-page downloadable booklet produced by the Office on Women's Health, U.S. Department of Health and Human Services.

Geddes Productions (instructional breastfeeding videos)
www.geddesproduction.com
Video titles include: *Breastfeeding after a Cesarean, The First Week,* and *Working Mother.*

International Lactation Consultant Association
www.ilca.org
A searchable directory to locate certified lactation consultants in your area.

La Leche League International
www.llli.org
Find a meeting near you, participate in a community message board, or read some of the useful information included on the LLL Web site.

Kathleen Huggins, *The Nursing Mother's Companion* (Boston: Harvard Common Press, 1999).
Excellent advice for the first few weeks of breastfeeding (and beyond). Troubleshoots common problems.

La Leche League, *The Womanly Art of Breastfeeding* (New York: Plume, 2004).
> In addition to solid advice about how to breastfeed your baby, this book encourages women to find support in other nursing mothers by attending such groups as La Leche League.

Massachusetts Breastfeeding Coalition
www.massbfc.org
> Web site offers breastfeeding tips in English, Spanish, Portugese, and French. Extensive collection of links to related breastfeeding advocacy organizations and other informative sites.

Breastfeeding Accessories

Make Your Own Nursing Pillow
www.sleepingbaby.net/jan/index.html?Baby/index.html
> If you know how to sew, this is a great project to make sure your nursing pillow is just the right size. Check out the other crafty activities offered on this Web site.

Medela
1-800-435-8316
www.medela.com
> Medela is the leader in breast pumps and accessories. Their "Personal Fit" line of breastshields offers pumping comfort for large-breasted women.

My Brest Friend
www.mybrestfriend.com
> Plus-size women rave about this nursing pillow for its fit and support (the pillow is secured to the waist with an adjustable strap for larger sizes).

Childbirth Preparation Classes

Each of these organizations teaches childbirth preparation classes stressing a nonmedicated approach to normal labor and delivery. The Web sites contain links to local instructors.

Birth Works, Inc.
  1-888-TO-BIRTH (1-800-862-4784)
  www.birthworks.org
  Classes provide physical and emotional preparation for childbirth
    and focus on relaxation techniques as primary form of pain
    relief.

The Bradley Method of Natural Childbirth
  American Academy of Husband-Coached Childbirth
  1-800-4-A-Birth (1-800-422-4784)
  www.bradleybirth.com
  Childbirth preparation classes stress the role of the partner as
    coach and primary support person.

HypnoBirthing Institute
  1-877-798-3286
  www.hypnobirthing.com
  Classes teach women relaxation and self-hypnotic techniques to
    reduce labor pain.

Lamaze International
  1-800-368-4404
  www.lamaze.org
  It's not just about breathing techniques! Lamaze classes teach
    movement and positioning, massage, relaxation, hydrotherapy,
    and the use of heat and cold to relieve labor pain.

Compulsive Overeating/ Binge Eating Disorder Support

Geneen Roth, *Breaking Free from Compulsive Eating* (New York:
Plume, 1993), *Feeding the Hungry Heart* (New York: Plume, 1993), and
When Food is Love (New York: Plume, 1992).
  For women who overeat to satisfy some kind emotional broken-
    ness, these books offer advice for how to finally make peace
    with yourself—and with food. Geneen draws upon her own
    experiences with compulsive overeating to create an extremely
    intimate and compelling portrayal of this disorder.

Eating Disorder Referral and Information Center
    www.edreferral.com
    Extensive links to local support groups and health-care profes-
        sionals specializing in eating disorders. Helpful fact sheet
        pages on binge eating disorder and overeating.

Overeaters Anonymous (12-Step Program)
    1-505-891-2664
    www.oa.org
    This Web site provides state-by-state and international meeting
        directories. Read more about what goes on at an OA meeting,
        and check out the inspirational stories written by some of the
        many helped through the OA program.

Domestic Violence

Call 911 or the local police department immediately if you ever fear that your partner is about to hurt you.

National Domestic Violence Hotline
    1-800-799-SAFE (1-800-799-7233)
    www.ndvh.org
    Callers receive crisis intervention, safety planning, information
        about domestic violence, and referrals to local service
        providers.

Doula Support

Each of the following organizations certifies doulas. Organization Web sites provide searchable databases to locate doulas in your area.

Association of Labor Assistants & Childbirth Educators (ALACE)
    1-617-441-2500/1-888-222-5223
    www.alace.org

Doulas of North America (DONA)
    1-888-788-DONA (1-888-788-3662)
    www.DONA.org

International Childbirth Education Association (ICEA)
    1-952-854-8660
    www.icea.org

Fertility

Robert Barbieri, Alice Domar, and Kevin Loughlin, *Six Steps to Increased Fertility* (New York: Fireside, 2000).
> Outlines a mind/body approach to fertility based on the Harvard Behavioral Medicine Program for Infertility.

Toni Wescheler, *Taking Charge of Your Fertility* (New York: Harper Collins, 2002).
> A comprehensive guide that is a must-read for any woman actively trying to get pregnant.

Big, Beautiful, and Trying to Conceive (message board)
> www.babycenter.com/bbs/1224440

Overweight and Trying to Conceive (support listserv)
> www.fertilityplus.org/bbw/otcc.html

RESOLVE
> 1-617-623-0744
> www.resolve.org
> Provides support and information for women and men experiencing infertility. The Web site contains links to local chapters.

Fitness

YMCA
> www.ymca.net
> There are more than 2,400 YMCAs in the United States, and many offer prenatal exercise and parent/baby classes. Use the Web site's search engine to find a YMCA near you.

Food Assistance

WIC Program
> www.fns.usda.gov/wic
> This Web site offers links to state agencies, WIC-approved farmers' markets, and information about WIC's commitment to breastfeeding support.

Gestational Diabetes

American Diabetes Association
   1-800-DIABETES (1-800-342-2383)
   www.diabetes.org/gestational-diabetes.jsp
   Organization dedicated to diabetes research and education. Their
      Web site offers links to recipes and meal planning.

American Diabetes Association, *Gestational Diabetes: What to Expect*
(Alexandria, VA: American Diabetes Association, 2001)
   Details the basics of how to care for yourself once you have been
      diagnosed with gestational diabetes.

Lois Jovanovic-Peterson, *Managing Your Gestational Diabetes* (New
York: Wiley, 1994).
   Detailed and reassuring information about what to expect when
      you are diagnosed with gestational diabetes.

Pregnant with Diabetes
   http://bbs.babycenter.com/board/pregnancy/pregcomplica-
      tions/1143961
   An active message board for women with gestational, Type I, or
      Type II diabetes.

Healthy Eating/ Nutrition

Walter Willet, *Eat, Drink and Be Healthy: The Harvard Medical School
Guide to Healthy Eating* (New York: Free Press, 2001).
   Promotes the Healthy Eating Pyramid as an alternative to the
      recently revised USDA food pyramid. Eye-opening information
      about how to choose healthy carbohydrates, fats, and proteins.
      Updated edition contains menu plans and recipes. Worth read-
      ing whether you are pregnant or not!

Catherine Jones and Rose Ann Hudson, *Eating for Pregnancy: An
Essential Guide to Nutrition with Recipes for the Whole Family* (New
York: Marlowe, 2003).
   Offers a wide variety of easy to prepare and nutritious dishes.

Judith Brown, *Nutrition and Pregnancy* (Los Angeles: Lowell House,
1998).
   Provides detailed information about basic nutrients, the increased

caloric demands of pregnancy and how what you eat helps ensure the delivery of a healthy, well-nourished baby.

Elizabeth Somer, *Nutrition for a Healthy Pregnancy* (New York: Holt, 2002).
   Offers healthy eating plans for preconception and pregnancy based on the latest research about prenatal nutrition.

March of Dimes
   www.marchofdimes.com
   Go to the "Pregnancy and Newborn Health Education Center" area of the Web site for information about good prenatal nutrition.

National Directory of Farmers' Markets
   www.ams.usda.gov/farmersmarkets/map.htm
   Find out when and where farmers' markets in your area take place.

Labor and Delivery

Barbara Harper, *Gentle Birth Choices* (Rochester, VT: Healing Arts Press, 2005).
   Details how to plan a meaningful and natural birth experience. The revised edition comes with a DVD showing a homebirth, waterbirth, vaginal birth after cesarean (VBAC), and birth with other children present.

Ina May Gaskin, *Ina May's Guide to Childbirth* (New York: Bantam, 2003).
   An inspiring guide to natural labor and delivery written by America's premier midwife and author of *Spiritual Midwifery*. Encourages women to trust their bodies during childbirth. Contains numerous birth stories and is a reassuring read for any woman as her due date approaches.

International Cesarean Awareness Network, Inc.
   1-800-686-ICAN (1-800-686-4336)
   www.ican-online.org
   ICAN's mission is to prevent medically unnecessary cesareans and promote VBAC through education and awareness. Their Web site offers empowering information about childbirth. If you have had a cesarean, check out the community bulletin boards to share your experiences with other women.

Polycystic Ovary Syndrome

Colette Harris, with Dr. Adam Carey, *PCOS: A Woman's Guide to Dealing with Polycystic Ovary Syndrome* (London: Thorsons, 2000).
  The first book to provide an in-depth look at PCOS. Offers a four-point plan to reduce symptoms.

Colette, Harris, with Theresa Cheung, *PCOS and Your Fertility* (Carlsbad, CA: Hay House, 2004).
  Written by two women with PCOS, this book includes everything you need to know about getting pregnant when you have PCOS.

Polycystic Ovary Syndrome Association (PCOSA)
  www.pcosupport.org
  Offers medical information and support communities. Their Web site provides a state-by-state database of "PCOSupport" chapters.

Soul Cysters
  www.soulcysters.com
  Online community of women with PCOS. Site created by former Consumer Health anchor for *CNN Headline News,* Kat Carney, after she was diagnosed with PCOS.

Postpartum Depression/Support

Postpartum Support International
  1-805-967-7636
  www.postpartum.net/index.html
  This Web site includes message boards, recovery stories, and a state-by-state directory of area support coordinators.

Depression After Delivery, Inc.
  www.depressionafterdelivery.com
  A national, nonprofit organization founded in 1985 by a woman who experienced postpartum depression. Site contains information about recognizing symptoms of PPD, support group directory, message boards, and recovery stories.

Preeclampsia Support/Bed Rest Resources

Denise M. Chism, *The High-Risk Pregnancy Sourcebook* (Los Angeles: Lowell House, 1998).
> Describes how women experiencing high-risk pregnancy can enhance their chances of having a healthy, full-term baby. Includes detailed information about preeclampsia and gestational hypertension.

Amy Tracy, *The Pregnancy Bed Rest Book: A Survival Guide for Expectant Mothers and Their Families* (New York: Berkley, 2001).
> Women on bed rest for any reason will find this book useful.

Preeclampsia Foundation
www.preeclampsia.org/
Information and support for women experiencing preeclampsia.

Sidelines National Support Network
www.sidelines.org
> Provides support for women and their families experiencing such complications as preeclampsia. The Web site offers active message board where women on bed rest can share their experiences.

Pregnancy, General Reading

American College of Obstetricians and Gynecologists, *Planning Your Pregnancy and Birth* (Washington, DC: ACOG, 2000).
> Clear and concise advice at your fingertips. The glossary of common obstetric terms is especially useful.

Ann Douglas, *The Mother of All Pregnancy Books* (New York: Wiley, 2002).
> Written in a fun-to-read style, this informative book is hard to put down.

Prenatal Health Care

American Academy of Family Physicians
1-800-274-2237
www.familydoctor.org
> Web site offers extensive health information on a variety of topics including pregnancy, childbirth, breastfeeding, and newborn

care. Search the database to locate family physicians in your local area (or call the toll-free number).

American College of Nurse-Midwives (ACNM)
1-202-728-9860
www.midwife.org
This Web site provides a wealth of information about why women should seriously consider receiving prenatal care from a certified nurse-midwife. Locate a CNM in your area with the searchable database.

American College of Obstetricians and Gynecologists
1-202-638-5577
www.acog.org
Mainly for the OB-GYN professional community, this Web site does contain a searchable database to help you locate an OB-GYN in your area.

Size-Friendly Healthcare Providers Database
www.cat-and-dragon.com/stef/Fat/ffp.html
State and local directories of size-friendly health-care professionals. Listings are submitted by patients or self-submitted by health providers who welcome working with plus-size people.

Quitting Smoking

A Breath of Fresh Air: Independence from Smoking
www.4woman.gov/stopsmoking
Run by the National Women's Health Information Center, this site contains extensive support and advice to help women stop smoking.

Great Start Quitline
1-866-66-START (1-866-667-8278)
Offers free one-on-one cessation counseling for pregnant smokers 24 hours/day. Callers can also request additional free quit smoking materials.

Smoke-Free Families
www.smokefreefamilies.org
Provides information and support for pregnant women to stop

smoking. Go to "Quit Now" area of Web site for practical advice and a state-by-state directory of smoking cessation resources for pregnant women.

Raising Healthy Families

Martha and William Sears, *The Baby Book* (New York: Little, Brown; 2003).
> Describes the basics of newborn care with the focus on "attachment parenting"—breastfeeding, baby-wearing, and sleeping with/near your baby as the best way to promote your baby's health and emotional development.

William Sears, *The Family Nutrition Book* (New York: Little, Brown; 1999).
> Lots of recipes and sound nutritional advice for every member of the family. This book is an indispensable part of any parenting library.

Allan Walker, with Courtney Humphries, *Eat, Play and Be Healthy: The Harvard Medical School Guide to Healthy Eating for Kids* (New York: McGraw-Hill, 2005).
> Scientifically based advice on nutritious eating for children. Lots of yummy recipes kids will love.

Mothering
> www.mothering.com
> A magazine devoted to giving mothers (and fathers) encouraging and helpful information about natural family living.

Women's Health

The Boston Women's Health Collective, *Our Bodies, Ourselves* (New York: Touchstone, 1998).
> The updated classic is still an empowering and relevant guide to women's health.

Susan Love, *The Breast Book* (New York: Perseus, 2000).
> Excellent reference on breast care.

National Women's Health Information Center
www.womenshealth.gov (or visit www.4women.gov)
Run by the U.S. government's Department of Health and Human
Services, this Web site contains a staggering array of health-
related information.

ACKNOWLEDGMENTS

WE EXTEND OUR gratitude and thanks to our agent, Agnes Birnbaum, for her unfailing support and wisdom about the publishing world. We thank Katie McHugh, our editor at Marlowe & Company, for her expertise in guiding this book through the publishing process, and Sue McCloskey, for so enthusiastically acquiring this project.

—*Cornelia van der Ziel* and *Jacqueline Tourville*

I WOULD LIKE to extend special thanks to Jacqueline Tourville for inviting me to collaborate in the writing of this book. Without her vision, this book would not have been possible.

I would like to thank the members of my family, especially my husband, Ken, for their support during the entire process. I would be remiss if I did not acknowledge my parents, Aldert and Jantina van der Ziel, who taught me the importance of perseverance and patience.

Jenny Weaver, an RN and lactation consultant in my office, was helpful in editing key portions of this book and in giving her unique perspective.

Lastly, I would like to thank my patients who have helped me become the doctor I am today. The sharing of their lives and medical care has introduced me to the diversity of the human experience.

—*Cornelia van der Ziel*

I sincerely thank the following people: Cornelia van der Ziel, for embracing this book and for her meticulous attention to detail; all the "sisters" who shared their stories during the writing of this book, especially the Winter Babes; my husband, Jason, who helped in countless ways; Claire, for showing up at the perfect time; my own sisters, Suzanne and Beth, for all their encouragement; my parents, Larry and Carol Tourville, for their love; Sylvia and Gloria, for sewing advice; Dave Schmelzer and VCF Cambridge; Krikor Bezjian, for the printer; Peter and Kristen Dame, for the camera; Alicia; Brian; Andrew; Patricia; Heidi; Zoe Gillis; Richard Goldwasser; Tim Myers, for helping me believe I could be a writer; and anyone and everyone who helped make the writing of this book the absolute blessing it has been.

—*Jacqueline Tourville*

INDEX

CPSIA information can be obtained at www.ICGtesting.com
Printed in the USA
LVOW12s0351290814

401293LV00002B/9/P